I0759113

THE PLANT-BASED REVOLUTION

DAVID SANDUA

INDEX

INTRODUCTION

The global food industry is experiencing a transformative shift towards plant-based diets and products, known as the plant-based revolution. With growing concerns about the environmental impact of animal agriculture, the rising prevalence of chronic diseases, and ethical considerations surrounding animal welfare, more and more people are adopting plant-based lifestyles. Plant-based diets primarily consist of fruits, vegetables, whole grains, legumes, nuts, and seeds, and exclude or minimize the consumption of animal products such as meat, dairy, and eggs. This dietary shift is not only reshaping the way individuals approach their daily meals but also influencing various industries, including food production, manufacturing, and agriculture. As this movement gains momentum, it is important to examine the reasons behind its popularity and its potential benefits for individuals and the planet. Through this essay, we will explore the underlying factors driving the plant-based revolution and the potential consequences it may have for individuals, public health, and the environment. By understanding the significance and implications of this trend, we can better comprehend the future of our food systems and make informed choices that contribute to a more sustainable and healthier planet.

DEFINITION OF PLANT-BASED DIETS

A plant-based diet can be defined as a nutritional approach that focuses mainly on consuming foods derived from plants, such as fruits, vegetables, whole grains, legumes, nuts, and seeds, while minimizing or completely eliminating the consumption of animal products. The emphasis is placed on the consumption of natural, unprocessed, and nutrient-dense plant foods that provide essential nutrients, including vitamins, minerals, fiber, antioxidants, and phytochemicals. Plant-based diets can take several forms, ranging from vegetarianism, which excludes meat but may include animal byproducts such as dairy and eggs, to veganism, which fully eliminates all animal products from the diet. There are variations and subcategories within plant-based diets, such as flexitarianism, which allows occasional or moderate consumption of animal products. The decision to adopt a plant-based diet is often driven by various factors, including health concerns, environmental sustainability, ethical considerations surrounding animal welfare, or simply a desire for a more diverse and flavorful culinary experience. Regardless of the specific motivation, adopting a plant-based diet has demonstrated numerous health benefits, including reduced risk of chronic diseases and improved overall well-being.

OVERVIEW OF THE PLANT-BASED REVOLUTION

This revolution in nutrition is characterized by a shift towards consuming plant-based foods, with an emphasis on whole, unprocessed fruits, vegetables, grains, legumes, and nuts. Plant-based diets have gained significant attention and popularity in recent years, as individuals are increasingly concerned about their health, the environment, and animal welfare. The benefits of adopting a plant-based diet are numerous and well-documented. These diets tend to be higher in fiber, vitamins, minerals, and antioxidants, and lower in saturated fats and cholesterol, compared to traditional animal-based diets. Research has shown that plant-based diets can reduce the risk of chronic diseases such as heart disease, obesity, type 2 diabetes, and certain types of cancers. The production of plant-based foods is more sustainable and environmentally friendly, requiring less water, land, and resources than animal agriculture. Choosing plant-based options can have positive implications for animal welfare, as it reduces the demand for animal products and supports more ethical and sustainable farming practices. The plant-based revolution represents a significant shift in the way we approach food and nutrition, with far-reaching implications for our well-being, the environment, and the ethical treatment of animals.

PURPOSE AND STRUCTURE OF THE ESSAY

The purpose and structure of an essay are crucial in effectively conveying the ideas and arguments addressed in the text. In the case of "The Plant-Based Revolution," the purpose is to examine the growing popularity of plant-based diets as a response to environmental and health concerns. This is achieved through a well-structured essay that begins with an introduction, providing a clear thesis statement and an overview of the topics that will be discussed. The body paragraphs then delve into the evidence and arguments supporting the benefits of plant-based diets, such as reduced carbon emissions, improved health outcomes, and ethical considerations. Each paragraph is dedicated to a specific aspect, organized in a logical manner that builds upon previous arguments and evidence. The essay employs effective transitions to ensure the smooth flow of ideas and to guide readers throughout the text. The purpose and structure of this essay allow for a comprehensive examination of the plant-based revolution, presenting a strong case for its merits and appealing to readers concerned about the environment and their well-being.

HISTORICAL CONTEXT OF PLANT-BASED EATING

In order to fully understand the contemporary relevance of plant-based eating, it is essential to examine its historical context. Plant-based diets have been an integral part of human nutrition for centuries, with evidence dating back to ancient civilizations such as the Greeks, Egyptians, and Chinese. The Pythagoreans, for instance, believed in the ethical and health benefits of abstaining from the consumption of meat and advocated for a plant-based lifestyle. Similarly, ancient Indian texts like the Ayurveda emphasize the consumption of plant-based foods for holistic well-being. In times of scarcity or religious observance, societies often turned to plant-based diets, as seen during periods of fasting in various religions. The advent of industrialization and the rise of animal agriculture during the late 19th and early 20th centuries heavily promoted meat consumption, leading to a decline in the prevalence of plant-based eating. In recent years, with growing concerns about the environmental impact of animal agriculture, health issues associated with excessive meat consumption, and ethical debates surrounding animal welfare, there has been a resurgence in the popularity of plant-based diets. Thus, understanding the historical context of plant-based eating provides valuable insight into the reasons behind its current revival and highlights its significance in contemporary society.

PLANT-BASED DIETS IN ANCIENT CULTURES

Another significant ancient culture that practiced plant-based diets was the ancient Greeks. Greek philosophers and physicians, such as Pythagoras and Hippocrates, advocated for the consumption of a predominantly plant-based diet. Pythagoras, known for his mathematical discoveries, believed in the concept of transmigration, where he taught that the human soul could be reincarnated into animals. Thus, he and his followers abstained from eating meat to avoid harming other souls. Hippocrates, often considered the father of medicine, promoted a plant-heavy diet for optimal health. He emphasized the importance of fruits, vegetables, and grains in maintaining a balanced and nutritious diet. Ancient Indian cultures, particularly those following Jainism and Buddhism, have long practiced plant-based diets. Jainism, one of the oldest religions in the world, promotes non-violence and compassion towards all living beings. As a result, Jains follow a strict vegetarian or vegan diet, avoiding the consumption of any animal products. Similarly, Buddhism espouses the principle of non-harming and encourages its followers to abstain from causing harm to animals through their diet. These ancient cultures recognized the benefits of a plant-based diet for their spiritual beliefs, as well as for their physical well-being.

EVOLUTION OF VEGETARIANISM AND VEGANISM

The evolution of vegetarianism and veganism can be attributed to the rise of ethical and environmental concerns. Many individuals have become aware of the inhumane treatment of animals in factory farming and the detrimental impact of animal agriculture on the environment. The documentary "Cowspiracy" brought these issues to the forefront, revealing the staggering environmental consequences of the meat industry, such as deforestation, greenhouse gas emissions, and water pollution. With this newfound knowledge, people have begun to question the morality and sustainability of consuming animal products. As a result, more individuals are opting for plant-based diets to minimize their contribution to animal suffering and environmental degradation. Beyond personal health and ethics, the plant-based movement has also gained momentum due to its association with social justice issues. Advocates argue that animal agriculture disproportionately affects disadvantaged communities, as factory farms are often located in low-income areas and contribute to air and water pollution. The evolution of vegetarianism and veganism can be seen as part of a broader movement towards promoting social and environmental wellbeing.

THE RESURGENCE OF PLANT-BASED EATING IN MODERN TIMES

One of the most significant factors contributing to the resurgence of plant-based eating in modern times is the growing awareness of the detrimental effects of animal agriculture on the environment. As the global climate crisis continues to escalate, more and more people are realizing the need to adopt sustainable practices in their daily lives. By choosing to follow a plant-based diet, individuals can significantly reduce their carbon footprint and mitigate the harmful effects of animal agriculture, such as deforestation and greenhouse gas emissions. The ethical concerns surrounding animal welfare have also played a crucial role in the growing popularity of plant-based eating. The exposure of inhumane practices within the meat and dairy industries has prompted many individuals to reevaluate their dietary choices and seek more compassionate alternatives. The health benefits associated with a plant-based diet have further contributed to its resurgence. Extensive research has shown that plant-based diets can help prevent and manage chronic illnesses, such as heart disease, diabetes, and obesity. As the evidence continues to mount, more individuals are turning to plant-based eating as a means to improve their overall well-being.

HEALTH MOTIVATIONS BEHIND PLANT-BASED DIETS

Plant-based diets have gained considerable attention in recent years due to the growing awareness of the health benefits associated with the consumption of plant-based foods. One of the primary motivations behind adopting a plant-based diet is the potential to improve overall health and reduce the risk of chronic diseases. Numerous studies have shown that diets rich in fruits, vegetables, whole grains, legumes, and nuts can lower the risk of conditions such as cardiovascular disease, type 2 diabetes, obesity, and certain types of cancer. Plant-based diets are typically low in saturated fat and cholesterol, while being high in fiber, antioxidants, and phytochemicals, which contribute to their health-promoting effects. Plant-based diets have been linked to weight loss, improved gut health, and a reduced likelihood of developing metabolic syndrome. Individuals who adhere to plant-based diets tend to have lower blood pressure, cholesterol levels, and markers of inflammation. The health benefits associated with plant-based diets make them an attractive dietary choice for individuals seeking to improve their well-being and reduce their risk of chronic diseases.

NUTRITIONAL BENEFITS OF PLANT-BASED FOODS

One cannot overlook the numerous nutritional benefits that plant-based foods provide. Plant-based diets are typically rich in vitamins, minerals, and antioxidants that are essential for maintaining optimal health. Fruits and vegetables are excellent sources of vitamin C, which plays a vital role in boosting the immune system and promoting healthy skin. Leafy greens such as spinach and kale are abundant in iron, a mineral crucial for transporting oxygen throughout the body. Plant-based foods are also a great source of fiber, which aids in digestion and helps prevent constipation. Research suggests that individuals following plant-based diets tend to have lower body mass indexes, reduced cholesterol levels, and a decreased risk of developing chronic diseases such as heart disease and certain types of cancer. This is mainly due to the absence of saturated fats and cholesterol found in animal-based products. Incorporating plant-based foods into one's diet can have tremendous health benefits and contribute to overall well-being.

PLANT-BASED DIETS AND CHRONIC DISEASE PREVENTION

Another significant benefit of plant-based diets is their potential role in chronic disease prevention. Numerous studies have shown that adopting a plant-based diet is associated with a reduced risk of developing chronic diseases such as heart disease, diabetes, and certain types of cancer. Research has consistently demonstrated that individuals who follow plant-based diets have lower levels of blood pressure, cholesterol, and body mass index compared to those who consume a high amount of animal products. This may be attributed to the fact that plant-based diets are typically high in fiber, antioxidants, and phytochemicals, all of which have been shown to have protective effects against chronic diseases. Plant-based diets are naturally low in saturated fats and cholesterol, which are known to contribute to the development of heart disease. The link between plant-based diets and chronic disease prevention is well-established, and it highlights the importance of considering plant-based diets as a viable option for maintaining optimal health and reducing the burden of chronic diseases.

WEIGHT MANAGEMENT AND PLANT-BASED EATING

Weight management is an important aspect of plant-based eating. Numerous studies have shown that individuals who follow a plant-based diet tend to have lower body mass index (BMI) and reduced rates of obesity compared to those who consume a diet high in animal products. This can be attributed to the fact that plant-based diets typically consist of foods that are low in calories and high in fiber, such as fruits, vegetables, whole grains, and legumes. These nutrient-dense foods provide a sense of fullness and satiety, leading to a decreased intake of calories and ultimately weight loss or weight maintenance. Plant-based diets are generally lower in saturated fats, which are found in high amounts in animal products. Excessive consumption of saturated fats has been linked to weight gain and an increased risk of chronic diseases such as heart disease and diabetes. Adopting a plant-based eating pattern can be an effective strategy for individuals looking to manage their weight and improve their overall health.

ENVIRONMENTAL MOTIVATIONS FOR CHOOSING PLANT-BASED

One of the most compelling motivations for choosing a plant-based diet is the desire to reduce the environmental impact of our food choices. Animal agriculture is a significant contributor to climate change, deforestation, and water pollution. The production of meat, dairy, and eggs requires vast amounts of land, water, and energy resources. According to recent studies, animal agriculture is responsible for approximately 14.5% of global greenhouse gas emissions, more than the entire transportation sector combined. Livestock production also plays a major role in deforestation, with vast areas of land being cleared to make way for grazing and growing animal feed crops. The excessive use of fertilizers and pesticides in animal agriculture contributes to water pollution and the destruction of aquatic ecosystems. By choosing plant-based foods, individuals can significantly reduce their carbon footprint and help mitigate climate change. Plant-based diets also require less land, water, and energy compared to animal-based diets, making them a more sustainable and environmentally friendly choice.

THE CARBON FOOTPRINT OF MEAT PRODUCTION

A major concern when discussing the plant-based revolution is the significant carbon footprint attributed to meat production. The livestock industry is responsible for a substantial amount of greenhouse gas emissions, deforestation, and water pollution. According to a report by the Food and Agriculture Organization of the United Nations, the livestock sector accounts for 14.5% of global greenhouse gas emissions, exceeding emissions from the transportation sector. The production and transport of feed crops, deforestation for grazing land, and methane emissions from enteric fermentation and manure management are some of the main contributors to the sector's environmental impact. The intensive use of water resources and contamination of water bodies with animal waste pose additional challenges. Transitioning towards a plant-based diet can significantly reduce the carbon footprint associated with food production. By eliminating animal agriculture, we can mitigate greenhouse gas emissions, reduce water usage, and conserve land resources. The adoption of plant-based diets not only benefits the environment but also offers a sustainable solution to feeding the growing global population.

WATER USAGE AND PLANT-BASED DIETS

Adopting a plant-based diet has significant implications for water usage. Industrial agriculture, which primarily produces animal-based foods, is a major consumer of water resources. In the United States, for instance, approximately 80% of the country's fresh water is used for agriculture (Environmental Protection Agency, 2021). This excessive water consumption is largely due to the vast amount of water needed to sustain animals raised for food, especially for the production of meat. In contrast, plant-based diets require significantly less water. It takes about 300 gallons of water to produce one pound of beef, compared to only 25 gallons of water for one pound of wheat (US Geological Survey, 2021). By shifting towards plant-based diets, individuals can help alleviate the burden on freshwater resources, especially in regions prone to water scarcity or drought. Thus, the promotion of plant-based diets is not only beneficial for human health and animal welfare, but also for the conservation and sustainable use of water resources.

BIODIVERSITY AND THE IMPACT OF ANIMAL AGRICULTURE

One major issue in the context of biodiversity is the considerable impact of animal agriculture. Animal agriculture has been identified as a significant driver of biodiversity loss and habitat destruction. The production of meat, dairy, and other animal-derived products requires large amounts of land for grazing, growing animal feed crops, and accommodating livestock. Consequently, forests and natural habitats are destroyed to create space for these activities. This destruction of habitats leads to the displacement and extinction of numerous plant and animal species that depend on these environments for survival. Animal agriculture contributes significantly to greenhouse gas emissions, which further exacerbates the effects of climate change and loss of biodiversity. The intensive practices utilized in animal farming, such as concentrated animal feeding operations (CAFOs), also pose a threat to wildlife populations and their ecosystems due to pollution and contamination of water bodies. To address this issue, it is crucial to transition towards more sustainable and plant-based food systems that reduce the reliance on animal agriculture and minimize the adverse effects it has on biodiversity.

ETHICAL CONSIDERATIONS IN DIET CHOICES

One important aspect of adopting a plant-based diet is the ethical consideration it entails. Many individuals are drawn to this dietary choice due to concerns about animal welfare and the environmental impacts of animal agriculture. By choosing to eat plant-based foods, individuals can actively contribute to the reduction of animal suffering and the conservation of natural resources. Factory farming practices, which often involve crowded and unsanitary conditions, can lead to the mistreatment and abuse of animals. The massive amounts of land, water, and feed required to sustain these operations contribute to deforestation, soil erosion, and water pollution. Adopting a plant-based diet represents a deliberate effort to align one's diet with their ethical values and contribute to a more sustainable and compassionate world. It is important to note that different individuals may have varying ethical considerations, and there remains ongoing debate about the most ethical dietary choices. Nonetheless, the growing popularity of plant-based diets reflects the increasing awareness and concern surrounding the ethical implications of food choices.

ANIMAL WELFARE CONCERNS

One of the key driving factors behind the plant-based revolution is the growing concern for animal welfare. As people become more aware of the conditions in which animals are raised for food production, there is a greater push for change. Factory farming practices that prioritize efficiency and profitability often result in cramped and unsanitary living conditions for animals. This not only compromises their physical health but also their mental well-being. Animals are social creatures that thrive in natural habitats and social structures, but in factory farms, they are stripped of their natural instincts and confined to tight spaces. The use of hormones, antibiotics, and other chemicals in animal agriculture has raised concerns about the potential health effects on humans. The plant-based movement offers a solution by promoting diets that rely on fruits, vegetables, whole grains, and legumes, eliminating the need to raise and slaughter animals. This shift not only reduces animal suffering but also contributes to a more sustainable and ethical food system.

ETHICAL FARMING PRACTICES

Ethical farming practices play a pivotal role in the plant-based revolution. As consumers become more conscious of the impact of their dietary choices on animal welfare and the environment, demand for ethically produced plant-based foods is on the rise. Ethical farming practices prioritize the well-being of animals, ensuring that they are provided with adequate living conditions, access to natural behaviors, and are treated humanely throughout their lives. These practices aim to minimize environmental harm by reducing greenhouse gas emissions, conserving water and land resources, and promoting biodiversity. The implementation of ethical farming practices also aligns with the principles of sustainability, as it fosters responsible food production that can meet the needs of the present generation without compromising the ability of future generations to meet their own needs. The adoption of ethical farming practices empowers consumers to make choices that promote animal welfare, environmental sustainability, and personal well-being, driving the plant-based revolution forward.

THE MORAL ARGUMENT FOR PLANT-BASED EATING

This emphasizes the ethical obligations of individuals towards animals and the environment. It is based on the belief that animals possess intrinsic value and deserve to be treated with respect and compassion. Advocates argue that consuming animal products perpetuates a system that causes immense suffering, as animals are often subjected to cruel farming practices and inhumane living conditions. By choosing to eat plants instead, individuals align their actions with their moral principles, promoting justice and compassion towards fellow beings. The industrial animal agriculture industry is a significant contributor to environmental degradation, including deforestation, pollution, and greenhouse gas emissions. By adopting a plant-based diet, individuals reduce their ecological footprint and contribute to a more sustainable future. This moral argument finds support in various philosophical and religious traditions, which promote the idea of stewardship and responsibility towards the environment and its inhabitants. The moral argument for plant-based eating provides a compelling case for conscious consumption, highlighting the profound impact our dietary choices can have on the well-being of animals and the planet.

THE SCIENCE OF PLANT-BASED NUTRITION

In order to truly understand the impact of plant-based nutrition, it is crucial to delve into the scientific basis underlying its benefits. Numerous studies have revealed the myriad ways in which a plant-based diet can positively affect human health. Research has consistently shown that individuals who consume plant-based diets tend to have lower rates of chronic diseases such as cardiovascular disease, obesity, and type 2 diabetes. This may be attributed to the fact that plant-based diets are typically rich in essential nutrients, such as fiber, vitamins, minerals, and antioxidants, all of which play a vital role in maintaining optimal health. The consumption of plant-based proteins, such as legumes, has been associated with a reduced risk of developing certain cancers. The environmental impact of a plant-based diet cannot be overlooked. The production of plant-based foods requires fewer resources, such as water and land, and produces fewer greenhouse gas emissions compared to animal agriculture. These scientific findings highlight the importance of embracing plant-based nutrition as a means of promoting both individual and planetary health.

MACRONUTRIENTS IN PLANT-BASED FOODS

Macronutrients are an essential component of plant-based foods and play a vital role in human nutrition. These nutrients include carbohydrates, proteins, and fats, each serving a unique purpose in the body. Carbohydrates are the primary energy source for our bodies and are abundant in plant-based foods such as fruits, vegetables, and whole grains. They are necessary for proper brain function and physical activity. Proteins, on the other hand, are the building blocks of life and are essential for the growth, repair, and maintenance of body tissues. Plant-based sources of protein include legumes, tofu, and tempeh, which offer a wide variety of amino acids necessary for optimal health. Fats are critical for the absorption of fat-soluble vitamins and provide energy during prolonged periods of exercise. Good sources of healthy fats in plant-based foods are avocados, nuts, and seeds. Understanding the importance of macronutrients in plant-based foods is crucial for individuals following a plant-based diet to ensure they meet their nutritional needs and maintain optimal health.

THE ROLE OF MICRONUTRIENTS AND PHYTOCHEMICALS

Micronutrients, such as vitamins and minerals, are essential for various body functions and play a significant role in maintaining overall health. Plant-based diets are abundant in these nutrients, particularly vitamins A, C, and E, as well as minerals like potassium, magnesium, and iron. These micronutrients have antioxidant properties that protect against oxidative stress, thereby preventing chronic diseases like cardiovascular disease and certain types of cancers. In addition to micronutrients, phytochemicals are bioactive compounds found exclusively in plants. These compounds have been widely studied for their potential health benefits. They act as antioxidants, anti-inflammatory agents, and even possess antimicrobial properties. Phytochemicals, such as flavonoids and carotenoids, have shown to play a protective role against chronic diseases, including diabetes and neurodegenerative disorders. Some studies suggest that certain phytochemicals might have anti-cancer properties. Incorporating a variety of plant-based foods into the diet ensures an adequate intake of micronutrients and phytochemicals, improving overall health and reducing the risk of chronic diseases.

DEBUNKING MYTHS ABOUT PLANT-BASED PROTEIN SOURCES

There are several myths surrounding plant-based protein sources that deserve to be debunked. The first myth is that plant-based proteins are not as complete as animal-based proteins. While it is true that plant-based proteins may lack specific essential amino acids, a well-balanced plant-based diet can easily provide all the necessary amino acids for optimal health. This can be achieved by consuming a variety of plant-based protein sources, such as legumes, grains, nuts, and seeds. Another common myth is that plant-based proteins are not as bioavailable as animal-based proteins. Studies have shown that the bioavailability of plant-based proteins can be enhanced by pairing them with complementary foods rich in certain amino acids or by using techniques such as fermentation or sprouting. The myth that plant-based proteins are less efficient for muscle building and recovery has been debunked by numerous studies demonstrating that plant-based athletes can achieve similar levels of strength and performance as their animal-based counterparts. It is important to challenge these myths and recognize the vast array of plant-based protein sources available that can support a healthy and sustainable diet.

PLANT-BASED DIETS AND GLOBAL HEALTH

Plant-based diets can have a substantial impact on global health. The consumption of animal products has been linked to various chronic diseases such as cardiovascular disease, type 2 diabetes, and certain types of cancer. On the other hand, plant-based diets, which are rich in fruits, vegetables, whole grains, legumes, and nuts, have been associated with a lower risk of these diseases. A shift towards more plant-based diets can help address the issue of global food security. Animal agriculture requires large amounts of land, water, and resources to sustain the production of meat, dairy products, and eggs. By adopting plant-based diets, individuals can significantly reduce their environmental footprint and contribute to the conservation of natural resources. Plant-based diets can also improve food accessibility and decrease the reliance on animal products, which are often more costly and less accessible for vulnerable populations. Promoting plant-based diets can serve as an effective strategy to enhance global health outcomes and contribute to a more sustainable and equitable food system.

ADDRESSING MALNUTRITION WITH PLANT-BASED OPTIONS

Plant-based diets, rich in a variety of fruits, vegetables, whole grains, legumes, and nuts, offer a wide array of essential nutrients needed for optimal health. These diets are particularly valuable in regions where access to animal-based products is limited or expensive. Plant-based options can help alleviate the burden on natural resources and mitigate the environmental impacts of industrialized animal agriculture. Plant-based diets have been associated with numerous health benefits, including reduced risk of chronic diseases like heart disease, obesity, and type 2 diabetes. It is crucial to emphasize the importance of a well-balanced and diverse plant-based diet to ensure adequate intake of all essential nutrients. Collaborative efforts among governments, international organizations, and local communities are necessary to promote the adoption of plant-based diets and provide education and resources on how to prepare nutritious plant-based meals. By prioritizing the incorporation of plant-based options into dietary recommendations and policies, we can actively address malnutrition and improve global health outcomes.

THE POTENTIAL FOR PLANT-BASED DIETS TO ALLEVIATE FOOD SCARCITY

As the global population continues to rise, strains on our food supply become increasingly apparent. Animal agriculture is a major contributor to this issue, as it requires vast amounts of land, water, and feed to sustain. By shifting towards plant-based diets, we can significantly reduce the demand for these resources and free up land and water for additional food production. Studies have shown that plant-based diets are more efficient in terms of land and water use, with some estimations suggesting a plant-based diet requires only 1/3 of the land and water compared to a meat-based diet. Plant-based diets can also address the issue of food waste. A substantial amount of food is lost or wasted during the production and processing of animal products. By reducing our reliance on animal agriculture, we can minimize food waste and increase food availability for those in need. By embracing plant-based diets, we have the opportunity to mitigate food scarcity and create a more sustainable food system for future generations.

THE ROLE OF PLANT-BASED DIETS IN GLOBAL HEALTH POLICY

There is a growing body of evidence that supports the benefits of plant-based diets in promoting good health and preventing chronic diseases. As a result, many countries are now adopting policies that promote the consumption of plant-based foods and discourage the consumption of animal products. In 2019, the EAT-Lancet Commission released a report that outlined a global planetary health diet, which recommended a significant reduction in the consumption of red meat and a substantial increase in the consumption of fruits, vegetables, legumes, and nuts. This report has influenced several countries to revise their dietary guidelines and incorporate more plant-based options. Organizations like the World Health Organization have also advocated for the inclusion of plant-based diets in global health policies, recognizing their potential to address not only individual health but also environmental sustainability and food security. The growing recognition of the role of plant-based diets in global health policy signifies a significant shift towards more sustainable and health-promoting food choices on a global scale.

THE ECONOMIC IMPACT OF THE PLANT-BASED TREND

The plant-based trend has had a significant economic impact on various sectors. One of the most notable consequences of this trend is the growth of the plant-based food industry. According to recent market research, the global plant-based meat market is projected to reach a value of $35.4 billion by 2027, with a compound annual growth rate of 15.8%. This growth can be attributed to several factors, including increased consumer awareness about the environmental and health benefits of plant-based diets, as well as the development of innovative plant-based products that closely resemble animal-based counterparts in taste and texture. The plant-based trend has also extended its influence to the fast-food industry. Many renowned fast-food chains have started incorporating plant-based options into their menus to cater to the growing demand for plant-based food. This trend is also driving innovation in the agriculture sector, with farmers exploring alternative crops and methods to meet the rising demand for plant-based ingredients. The economic impact of the plant-based trend is multifaceted and has the potential to reshape various industries.

COST COMPARISON BETWEEN PLANT-BASED AND MEAT-BASED DIETS

A significant factor that contributes to the popularity of plant-based diets is the cost comparison between plant-based and meat-based diets. It has been widely acknowledged that a plant-based diet, consisting of whole grains, legumes, fruits, and vegetables, can be more affordable compared to a diet dominated by animal products. According to a study conducted by the Journal of Hunger & Environmental Nutrition, researchers discovered that plant-based diets tend to be significantly cheaper than meat-based diets. The study found that the cost per serving of protein was much lower for plant-based foods such as lentils, beans, and tofu compared to animal-based options like beef and chicken. Plant-based diets emphasize consuming whole and unprocessed foods, which are often more economical in the long run. In contrast, animal-based products, especially high-quality sources of meat and dairy, can be relatively expensive. These findings highlight the potential economic benefits of adopting a plant-based diet, making it a more accessible and affordable option for individuals pursuing dietary changes.

THE EFFECT ON THE AGRICULTURE INDUSTRY

The plant-based revolution is having a profound impact on the agriculture industry. With the increasing demand for plant-based foods, farmers are shifting their focus and investing in crops such as legumes, grains, and vegetables. This shift is not only driven by changing consumer preferences but also by the realization that plant-based agriculture is more sustainable and environmentally friendly than traditional animal agriculture. By reducing the reliance on animal products, farmers can minimize the need for land, water, and feed, leading to a more efficient use of resources. The cultivation of plant-based crops can help mitigate the negative environmental effects associated with livestock farming, such as greenhouse gas emissions and pollution from manure. As a result of this shift, the agriculture industry is witnessing a transformation in farming practices, with more farmers adopting organic and regenerative farming techniques to meet the growing demand for plant-based foods. The plant-based revolution is driving a positive change in the agriculture industry, promoting sustainable practices and providing opportunities for farmers to diversify their crops and meet the evolving needs of consumers.

JOB CREATION IN THE PLANT-BASED FOOD SECTOR

As more people embrace a plant-based lifestyle, there is a growing demand for plant-based food products. This demand has led to the emergence of various plant-based food companies, ranging from startups to well-established brands. These companies require a skilled workforce to handle areas such as food processing, product development, marketing, and distribution. Consequently, job opportunities have been created for individuals interested in pursuing careers in the plant-based food sector. The plant-based revolution has also triggered the need for research and development in this field. Scientists and researchers are constantly working towards creating new and innovative plant-based alternatives to traditional animal-based products. This has expanded the scope for employment in scientific research and development roles. As the plant-based food sector continues to grow, it also creates indirect employment opportunities in related industries such as agriculture, packaging, and logistics. Thus, the growth of the plant-based food sector not only provides consumers with healthier and environmentally friendly food choices but also contributes to job creation and economic development.

THE RISE OF PLANT-BASED FOOD PRODUCTS

While the plant-based movement has gained significant momentum in recent years, it is important to note that this rise did not happen overnight. The growing interest in plant-based food products can be attributed to a variety of factors. First and foremost, there has been a surge in consumer awareness and concern about the environmental impact of animal agriculture. As individuals become more educated about the detrimental effects of meat and dairy production on climate change, deforestation, and water pollution, many are opting for plant-based alternatives as a way to minimize their ecological footprint. The rise of social media and the spread of information have played a crucial role in popularizing plant-based diets. Influencers, celebrities, and health experts have taken to online platforms to advocate for plant-based lifestyles, showcasing the health benefits and delicious recipes associated with this dietary choice. Advancements in food technology have made it easier than ever to create and market plant-based food products that mimic the taste and texture of traditional animal-derived foods. Products such as veggie burgers, plant-based milks, and vegan cheeses are now widely available in supermarkets and restaurants, catering to the growing demand for plant-based options.

INNOVATION IN PLANT-BASED MEAT ALTERNATIVES

With growing concerns about the environmental impact of traditional meat production and the rising demand for healthier and more sustainable options, the development of plant-based meats has witnessed significant advancements. The innovative strategies employed by food companies have resulted in the creation of products that closely resemble the taste, texture, and nutritional profile of animal-based meats. Through the utilization of cutting-edge technologies, such as genetic engineering and 3D printing, scientists and researchers have been able to experiment with various plant-based ingredients, and manipulate their characteristics to mimic the sensory experience of consuming meat. The use of advanced cooking techniques, like sous-vide and high-pressure processing, further enhances the texture and flavor of these alternatives. Innovative packaging designs and marketing strategies have also contributed to the success of these plant-based alternatives, attracting a wider consumer base. The continuous evolution and improvement of plant-based meat alternatives through innovation have undoubtedly played a critical role in driving the plant-based revolution forward.

THE GROWTH OF DAIRY-FREE MILK AND CHEESE PRODUCTS

The demand for alternatives to traditional dairy products has skyrocketed in recent years due to various factors, including health concerns, environmental awareness, and animal welfare considerations. As a response to this growing demand, numerous companies have emerged, offering a wide range of plant-based milk and cheese alternatives made from sources such as soy, almonds, cashews, and oats. These products offer a similar taste and texture to their dairy counterparts while being free from lactose and cholesterol. They are often fortified with essential nutrients such as calcium, vitamin D, and vitamin B12, making them a suitable choice for individuals looking to maintain a balanced diet. The availability and variety of dairy-free milk and cheese products have expanded to the point where they are now easily accessible in mainstream grocery stores, coffee shops, and restaurants. As consumers become increasingly health-conscious and environmentally aware, the trend towards dairy-free alternatives is likely to continue growing, ultimately transforming the way we view and consume dairy products.

EXPANSION OF PLANT-BASED OPTIONS IN RESTAURANTS AND FAST FOOD

With the ever-increasing popularity of plant-based diets, there has been a significant expansion of plant-based options in restaurants and fast-food chains. Consumers are becoming more conscious about their health and the environmental impact of their food choices, leading to a shift towards plant-based alternatives. Restaurateurs and fast-food chains have recognized this growing demand and are adapting their menus to cater to this demographic. Many restaurants now offer a wide range of plant-based options, including vegetarian and vegan dishes that are not only healthy but also delicious. Fast-food chains, typically known for their meat-centric menus, have also introduced plant-based alternatives, such as veggie burgers and plant-based chicken substitutes. This expansion of plant-based options is not only beneficial for individuals following plant-based diets, but it also encourages others to incorporate more plant-based foods into their meals, thereby contributing to a more sustainable and eco-friendly food system. As the plant-based revolution continues to gain momentum, it is expected that the expansion of plant-based options in restaurants and fast-food chains will only continue to grow, accommodating the increasing demand for plant-based alternatives in the market.

CONSUMER BEHAVIOR AND PLANT-BASED DIETS

Consumer behavior plays a significant role in the growing popularity of plant-based diets. As more people become aware of the environmental and health benefits associated with consuming less animal products, they are increasingly adopting plant-based eating patterns. One key aspect of consumer behavior in relation to plant-based diets is the desire for ethical consumption. Many individuals are now more conscious of the negative impact that animal agriculture has on animal welfare and the environment, and they seek to align their dietary choices with their values. Consumer behavior also plays a role in the perception and acceptance of plant-based alternatives. As companies continue to develop and market plant-based products that mimic the taste, texture, and appearance of animal-derived foods, consumers are more likely to try and adopt these products. The rise of social media platforms and online communities related to plant-based eating have helped to create a sense of community and support for those adopting this dietary approach. Consumer behavior is driving the plant-based revolution by influencing dietary choices, promoting ethical consumption, and fostering acceptance of plant-based alternatives.

DEMOGRAPHICS OF PLANT-BASED DIET ADOPTERS

A key aspect of studying the plant-based revolution is understanding the demographics of those who adopt a plant-based diet. Research suggests that there is a wide range of individuals who choose to follow this dietary lifestyle. In terms of age, it has been found that younger generations, particularly millennials and Generation Z, are more likely to adopt a plant-based diet compared to older generations. This may be due to increased awareness of environmental and ethical concerns related to animal agriculture, as well as a desire to improve personal health. Studies have shown that women are more likely to embrace a plant-based diet than men. This gender disparity could be attributed to societal pressures for women to embrace healthier eating habits and a greater inclination towards compassion for animals. Socioeconomic factors also play a role, with higher income and education levels being associated with a higher likelihood of adopting a plant-based diet. It is important to note that as plant-based diets become more mainstream, they are attracting individuals from a variety of demographic backgrounds. Thus, understanding the demographics of plant-based diet adopters is crucial for assessing the potential impact of this dietary shift on society.

MARKETING AND THE INFLUENCE ON CONSUMER CHOICES

Marketing plays a pivotal role in influencing consumer choices, particularly in relation to the plant-based revolution. As consumer interest in healthier and more sustainable lifestyles continues to grow, companies have capitalized on this trend by promoting plant-based products through strategic marketing efforts. In order to sway consumer preferences, marketers employ various tactics such as persuasive messaging, influential endorsement, and creative branding. Through the use of compelling advertisements and social media campaigns, companies are able to highlight the benefits of plant-based alternatives, such as their positive impact on personal health, animal welfare, and the environment. Collaborations with well-known influencers and celebrities who advocate for plant-based diets further reinforce the desirability of these products. By utilizing these marketing strategies, companies are able to shape consumer attitudes and behaviors, ultimately driving the demand for plant-based options. It is essential for consumers to critically evaluate the information presented to them and ensure that their choices align with their personal values and wellness goals. With the increasing influence of marketing in shaping consumer choices, individuals must exercise a discerning eye in order to make informed decisions and contribute to the sustainability and well-being of our planet.

THE ROLE OF SOCIAL MEDIA IN THE PLANT-BASED MOVEMENT

Over the past decade, social media platforms have become powerful tools for spreading information, raising awareness, and mobilizing communities around various causes. The plant-based movement, which advocates for a shift towards animal-free diets and a more sustainable food system, has greatly benefitted from social media's reach and influence. Platforms such as Instagram, Facebook, and YouTube have allowed activists, influencers, and organizations to share compelling photos, videos, and personal stories that highlight the benefits of plant-based diets. The use of hashtags like #plantbased, #vegan, and #meatlessmonday has facilitated the creation of online communities, connecting individuals from all walks of life who share a common interest in plant-based living. This online support network provides information, guidance, and motivation, making it easier for individuals to adopt and maintain a plant-based lifestyle. Social media has played a crucial role in challenging mainstream narratives about food and nutrition, exposing the environmental and ethical consequences of animal agriculture, and providing a platform for marginalized voices within the plant-based movement. Social media has revolutionized the way information is disseminated and has significantly influenced the growth and impact of the plant-based movement.

CHALLENGES OF TRANSITIONING TO PLANT-BASED EATING

Transitioning to a plant-based eating lifestyle poses a number of challenges for individuals. One significant challenge is the lack of knowledge and understanding about plant-based nutrition. Many people have grown up with the belief that a balanced diet includes meat, dairy, and other animal products. They may be unfamiliar with the nutritional requirements of a plant-based diet and how to properly meet them. There is a misconception that plant-based eating is expensive and inaccessible. While some plant-based products can be pricier than their animal-based counterparts, there are plenty of affordable plant-based options available. Another challenge is the social aspect of transitioning to plant-based eating. Many social gatherings and events revolve around food, and it can be difficult to navigate these situations when following a plant-based diet. It may be necessary to plan ahead and communicate dietary restrictions to hosts in order to ensure that suitable options are available. Transitioning to plant-based eating requires education, planning, and adaptability to overcome these challenges and make sustainable dietary choices.

OVERCOMING TASTE PREFERENCES AND HABITS

For many individuals, taste preferences are deeply ingrained and influenced by cultural and societal norms. The consumption of animal products has become so deeply rooted in our eating habits that it may seem daunting to relinquish these preferences. By exposing ourselves to new flavors and experimenting with plant-based alternatives, we can begin to overcome these taste preferences. It is important to approach this shift with an open mind and a willingness to try new things. Exploring a variety of spices, herbs, and different cooking techniques can help enhance the flavors of plant-based dishes and make them more enjoyable. It is crucial to recognize that our taste preferences are not fixed and can change over time. By consistently exposing ourselves to plant-based foods, our taste buds will adapt, and we may find ourselves beginning to appreciate and even prefer these alternatives. Overcoming taste preferences and habits is an ongoing process that requires patience and persistence but can ultimately lead to a successful transition to a plant-based diet.

ACCESSIBILITY AND AVAILABILITY OF PLANT-BASED FOODS

As demand for plant-based products continues to rise, food manufacturers and retailers have responded by expanding their offerings of plant-based options. This means that consumers now have more choices and easier access to a wide variety of plant-based foods. The increase in availability of plant-based options has not been limited to specialty stores or health food markets; it has reached mainstream supermarkets and restaurants as well. This increased accessibility has made it easier for individuals to adopt plant-based diets, regardless of their location or income level. The rise of online shopping platforms has made it even more convenient for consumers to order plant-based products directly to their doorsteps. This availability and accessibility of plant-based foods has contributed greatly to the overall acceptance and adoption of plant-based diets, as individuals now have more opportunities to incorporate healthy, sustainable, and ethical food choices into their lifestyles.

NUTRITIONAL CONCERNS AND EDUCATION

While a plant-based diet can provide many health benefits, it is crucial to ensure that individuals are adequately meeting their nutritional needs. One concern often raised is the adequacy of protein intake. Research has shown that plant-based diets can easily meet protein requirements by including a variety of plant-based protein sources such as legumes, tofu, tempeh, and quinoa. Vitamin B12 is a nutrient that is primarily found in animal products and is essential for maintaining nerve function and producing DNA. Individuals following a plant-based diet need to ensure they obtain adequate amounts through fortified foods or supplements. Education is also necessary to ensure that individuals understand the importance of balanced meal planning and the inclusion of essential nutrients like iron, calcium, and omega-3 fatty acids. By providing accurate and evidence-based information about the plant-based diet, individuals can make informed decisions about their dietary choices and optimize their nutritional status.

THE ROLE OF GOVERNMENTS IN THE PLANT-BASED MOVEMENT

Governments play a significant role in the plant-based movement by implementing policies and regulations that promote the adoption of plant-based diets. They have the power to influence individuals' dietary choices through educational campaigns, taxes on animal products, and subsidies for plant-based alternatives. By raising awareness about the environmental and health benefits of plant-based diets, governments can encourage citizens to make more sustainable and health-conscious food choices. They can support research and development in plant-based agriculture, providing funding and incentives to farmers who transition from animal-based agriculture to plant-based practices. Governments can also collaborate with the food industry to introduce labeling standards that clearly identify plant-based products, making it easier for consumers to choose sustainable options. Governments can promote plant-based diets in public institutions, such as schools, hospitals, and correctional facilities, ensuring that nutritious and plant-based meals are accessible to all. In summary, by actively supporting the plant-based movement, governments can foster a more sustainable, equitable, and healthy food system for present and future generations.

POLICY INITIATIVES PROMOTING PLANT-BASED DIETS

Governments and organizations around the world are recognizing the potential benefits of transitioning to a plant-based diet for both human health and environmental sustainability. One notable policy initiative is the implementation of nutrition guidelines that emphasize the consumption of plant-based foods. In the United States, the Dietary Guidelines for Americans recommend the inclusion of a variety of fruits, vegetables, legumes, and whole grains in daily meals. Some countries have introduced meat reduction or meat-free days as part of their public health campaigns. These initiatives aim to increase public awareness about the impact of meat consumption on health and the environment, and to encourage individuals to opt for plant-based alternatives. Policy initiatives promoting plant-based diets can also extend to schools and hospitals. By incorporating more plant-based options in cafeterias and patient menus, these institutions contribute to the normalization and accessibility of plant-based choices. These policy initiatives play a crucial role in fostering a plant-based revolution by shaping public attitudes and behaviors towards more sustainable and healthy dietary habits.

SUBSIDIES AND THEIR IMPACT ON FOOD CHOICES

Subsidies play a significant role in shaping food choices and consumption patterns. In the context of the plant-based revolution, the impact of subsidies on food choices becomes crucial. Subsidies offered to traditional animal-based agricultural practices, such as the production of meat and dairy, distort market prices and make these products more affordable compared to plant-based alternatives. Consequently, consumers are incentivized to opt for animal products, which are often high in fat, cholesterol, and unsustainable in terms of environmental impact. The pervasive influence of subsidies contributes to the prevalence of a standard Western diet that has been associated with various health issues and climate change. In contrast, the limited support provided to plant-based alternatives affects their affordability and accessibility. Increased subsidies for plant-based foods could make them more competitive in the market and potentially shift food consumption patterns towards healthier and more sustainable options. By redirecting subsidies towards plant-based agriculture, policymakers have the opportunity to create a more equitable food system that promotes both personal and planetary well-being.

PUBLIC HEALTH CAMPAIGNS AND EDUCATION

These campaigns aim to raise awareness about the detrimental effects of a meat-centric diet on personal health and the environment, while highlighting the positive impact of embracing plant-based alternatives. Through educational initiatives, individuals can be informed about the nutritional composition of plant-based foods and how they can fulfill dietary requirements. Public health campaigns work to debunk common myths surrounding plant-based diets, such as the notion that they lack sufficient protein or other essential nutrients. By providing accurate information and dispelling misconceptions, these initiatives empower individuals to make informed decisions about their dietary choices. Public health campaigns often collaborate with schools and other educational institutions to incorporate plant-based nutrition into the curriculum, thereby fostering healthy habits from a young age. These campaigns and education efforts have the potential to inspire a shift towards plant-based diets, leading to improved individual health and contributing to a sustainable future for all.

THE INTERSECTION OF PLANT-BASED DIETS AND CULTURE

In today's increasingly globalized world, the intersection of plant-based diets and culture has become a topic of immense interest and significance. As individuals become more aware of the impact of their dietary choices on not only their personal health but also the environment, the adoption of plant-based diets has gained momentum. It is crucial to recognize that cultural factors play a pivotal role in shaping dietary practices and preferences. Different cultures have distinct culinary traditions and food norms rooted in historical, social, and religious contexts. Thus, when discussing the adoption of plant-based diets, it is imperative to acknowledge and respect cultural diversity. Cultural assimilation and globalization have led to the fusion of cuisines and the incorporation of plant-based elements into diverse culinary traditions. This intersection has allowed for the development of innovative and diverse plant-based dishes that cater to different cultural tastes while promoting sustainability and health. Thus, the intersection of plant-based diets and culture presents an opportunity for fostering inclusivity, promoting sustainable living, and sparking culinary creativity on a global scale.

PLANT-BASED EATING IN DIFFERENT CULTURAL CONTEXTS

These cultural differences in plant-based eating reflect the diverse ways in which people interact with and value food. In many Asian cultures, such as Japan and China, plant-based diets have long been a central part of traditional cuisine. These diets often emphasize vegetables, legumes, and grains, while minimizing the consumption of meat and animal products. Meanwhile, in certain African and Middle Eastern cultures, plant-based eating is also an integral part of the culinary tradition. Traditional dishes such as falafel and hummus in the Middle East, and injera and lentil stews in Ethiopia, are all centered around plant-based ingredients. On the other hand, in Western cultures, the emphasis on meat and animal products has historically been more pronounced, although this is shifting as plant-based eating gains popularity. The cultural context in which plant-based eating takes place shapes people's attitudes and practices towards food, as well as their beliefs and values regarding health, ethics, and sustainability. Understanding the cultural nuances of plant-based eating is essential for promoting the acceptance and adoption of plant-based diets across different societies.

TRADITIONAL CUISINES ADAPTING TO PLANT-BASED TRENDS

There has been a notable shift towards plant-based diets and lifestyles. Traditional cuisines, known for their rich meat and dairy-based dishes, are now adapting to these plant-based trends. Many traditional cultures have a long history of incorporating plant-based ingredients into their dishes, making it easier for them to adjust to this new demand. In Asian cuisine, tofu, soy milk, and a wide variety of vegetables have always played a significant role. Chefs are now exploring innovative ways to transform traditional meat-centric dishes into plant-based alternatives. Plant-based burgers, sausages, and even seafood are appearing on menus, utilizing ingredients such as mushrooms, lentils, and jackfruit to mimic the taste and texture of the original dishes. This adaptation not only caters to the growing demand for plant-based options but also provides an opportunity for traditional cuisines to evolve and stay relevant. This transition towards plant-based alternatives in traditional cuisines is not only a response to changing dietary preferences but also reflects a larger shift towards sustainable and environmentally friendly practices in the food industry.

CULTURAL RESISTANCE TO PLANT-BASED DIETS

The deep-rooted cultural attachment to meat consumption is multifaceted and can be observed in various societies around the world. One element of this resistance is the perception that plant-based diets are nutritionally deficient, leading to concerns about adequate protein intake, iron, and other essential vitamins and minerals. These misconceptions are often perpetuated by mainstream media and the meat industry, which have a vested interest in maintaining the status quo. Cultural traditions and norms play a crucial role in shaping dietary choices. In many cultures, meat is closely associated with wealth, power, and celebration, making it challenging to shift behaviors and mentality. The perception of plant-based diets as "bland" or "restrictive" can deter individuals from adopting such lifestyles. The cultural resistance to plant-based diets underscores the need for education and awareness campaigns that dispel myths about the adequacy of plant-based nutrition and promote the wide variety and flavors of plant-based foods. Only through dismantling these ingrained cultural attitudes can the plant-based revolution truly thrive.

THE PSYCHOLOGICAL ASPECTS OF EATING HABITS

Understanding the psychological aspects of eating habits is crucial in analyzing the impact of the plant-based revolution. A person's relationship with food is deeply rooted in their emotions, beliefs, and learned behaviors, all of which play a significant role in determining their dietary choices. Psychologists have identified various factors that influence eating habits, including stress, emotional well-being, self-control, and social environment. Stress, for instance, has been found to lead to emotional eating, whereby individuals consume food to cope with negative emotions. This often results in the consumption of unhealthy, high-calorie foods. Emotional well-being is closely tied to eating habits; individuals in a positive emotional state tend to make healthier food choices, while those experiencing negative emotions are more likely to seek comfort in unhealthy foods. Individuals with high self-control are more likely to adhere to healthier eating habits, as they are better able to resist tempting but unhealthy food options. The social environment, including family and peer influences, greatly shape an individual's eating habits by reinforcing certain food preferences and dietary norms. Considering these psychological aspects is vital in understanding the potential challenges and motivations people face when transitioning to a plant-based diet.

EMOTIONAL CONNECTIONS TO FOOD AND MEAT CONSUMPTION

Many people have strong attachments to the taste, texture, and memories associated with consuming meat. The act of cooking and sharing meat-centered meals can hold cultural and social significance, forging deeper bonds within families and communities. The consumption of meat can evoke feelings of comfort, satiation, and nostalgia due to its prevalence in traditional dishes and holiday celebrations. These emotional attachments make it challenging for individuals to transition to a plant-based diet, as they fear losing those familiar sensory experiences and social connections. Societal norms and expectations often reinforce the emotional connection to meat consumption, as it remains a symbol of wealth, power, and masculinity. Consequently, individuals who choose to adopt a plant-based diet may face resistance and scrutiny from those who view meat consumption as an inherent part of their identity. Acknowledging the emotional connections to food and meat consumption is crucial in understanding the barriers individuals encounter when seeking alternatives, fostering a more empathetic approach towards encouraging the plant-based revolution.

COGNITIVE DISSONANCE AND ETHICAL EATING

Cognitive dissonance refers to the psychological discomfort individuals experience when they hold two conflicting beliefs or when their beliefs are incongruent with their actions. In the context of ethical eating, cognitive dissonance may arise when individuals are aware of the ethical implications of their food choices but continue to consume meat and animal-based products. Despite having knowledge about the negative impacts of the meat industry on the environment, animal welfare, and human health, individuals often struggle to align this knowledge with their eating habits. This cognitive dissonance can be attributed to various factors, including societal norms, cultural traditions, and personal habits. Ethical eating requires individuals to confront and resolve this cognitive dissonance by adopting more sustainable and compassionate food choices. Altering deeply ingrained eating behaviors can be challenging, especially when they are deeply intertwined with an individual's identity and sense of belonging. Overcoming cognitive dissonance related to ethical eating involves a process of reevaluating one's beliefs, educating oneself on the ethical and environmental consequences of food choices, and actively seeking alternatives that align with one's values and principles. The journey towards ethical eating requires individuals to confront the discomfort of cognitive dissonance and make conscious decisions that promote the well-being of animals, the environment, and themselves.

THE IMPACT OF SOCIETAL NORMS ON DIET CHOICES

Societal norms play a significant role in shaping individuals' diet choices. In contemporary society, the dominant paradigm often prioritizes convenience, taste, and social acceptance over health and sustainability. As a result, individuals frequently succumb to the pressures of conforming to unhealthy dietary practices. Fast food chains, for instance, are pervasive in popular culture and are often associated with convenience and affordability. This societal acceptance and normalization of fast food consumption perpetuate unhealthy eating habits. The influence of advertising and marketing campaigns cannot be underestimated. Companies strategically promote unhealthy, highly processed, and animal-based products, appealing to consumers' desires and preferences. The constant exposure to advertisements and societal pressure create a sense of normalcy around unhealthy food choices, making it difficult for individuals to resist. Cultural and social norms also shape diet choices. In many societies, meat and dairy products are traditionally associated with wealth and social status, while plant-based alternatives may be viewed as unconventional or even rebellious. Consequently, individuals may face resistance and criticism when opting for a plant-based diet, reinforcing the dominance of societal norms and making it challenging to deviate from them. Societal norms exert a powerful influence on individuals' diet choices, deterring them from embracing healthier, more sustainable options.

THE ROLE OF CHEFS AND CULINARY EXPERTS

Chefs and culinary experts play a crucial role in the plant-based revolution. As society becomes more conscious of the environmental impacts and health benefits associated with adopting a plant-based diet, these professionals have the opportunity to innovate and create culinary experiences that challenge conventional notions of taste and flavor. Their expertise and creativity are essential in developing plant-based dishes that appeal to all palates, including those who are skeptical about giving up meat. By incorporating a variety of ingredients and techniques, chefs can showcase the vast possibilities of plant-based cuisine, demonstrating that it can be vibrant, diverse, and satisfying. They can educate the public about the nutritional benefits of plant-based eating and dispel any misconceptions about the lack of protein or flavor in these types of diets. Chefs and culinary experts also have the power to influence the larger food industry by promoting sustainable sourcing practices and advocating for plant-based options in restaurants and food establishments. Their role extends beyond the kitchen as they become ambassadors for the plant-based movement, inspiring others to make conscious food choices that benefit both their health and the planet.

INNOVATIONS IN PLANT-BASED COOKING

There has been a surge of innovations in plant-based cooking, revolutionizing the way people approach vegetarian and vegan cuisine. With increasing concerns over health, animal welfare, and sustainability, individuals and chefs alike are seeking to create dishes that not only cater to different dietary preferences but also provide a delightful gastronomic experience. One notable innovation in plant-based cooking is the development of meat substitutes that closely resemble the taste and texture of meat. Companies like Beyond Meat and Impossible Foods have successfully created plant-based alternatives that have gained substantial popularity among both vegans and non-vegans. Another remarkable innovation in plant-based cooking is the use of unconventional ingredients to create unique flavor profiles. Chefs are now experimenting with ingredients like jackfruit, tempeh, and seitan to add meaty textures and flavors to their dishes. Advancements in food technology have paved the way for the creation of plant-based dairy products like cheese and ice cream that convincingly mimic their animal-based counterparts. These innovations in plant-based cooking not only challenge traditional culinary practices but also offer more sustainable and ethical alternatives to traditional meat and dairy products.

PROFESSIONAL TRAINING FOR PLANT-BASED CUISINE

Chefs and culinary professionals are now seeking specialized education and training programs to enhance their skills in creating flavorful and innovative plant-based dishes. One example of such a program is the Plant-Based Culinary Arts Program offered at the Natural Gourmet Institute in New York City. This program teaches students how to incorporate whole, plant-based foods into their cooking, while also providing them with a foundation in nutrition and food science. Students learn techniques for preparing dishes that showcase the natural flavors and textures of plant-based ingredients, as well as methods for creating plant-based versions of classic dishes. The program emphasizes the importance of sustainability, ethical sourcing of ingredients, and the role of plant-based cuisine in combating climate change. By providing professional training in plant-based cuisine, programs like the one offered at the Natural Gourmet Institute are equipping chefs with the knowledge and skills they need to meet the growing demand for plant-based options in restaurants and other food establishments.

CELEBRITY CHEFS AND THE PROMOTION OF PLANT-BASED DIETS

Celebrity chefs have played a significant role in promoting plant-based diets by showcasing the versatility and culinary appeal of plant-based foods. There has been a surge of celebrity chefs, such as Jamie Oliver and Gordon Ramsay, who have embraced plant-based cooking and advocated for its benefits. These chefs utilize their platforms to create mouth-watering plant-based recipes and share them with their audience, thereby challenging the stereotype that vegan or vegetarian food is bland or tasteless. By presenting plant-based meals as exciting and delicious alternatives, celebrity chefs have encouraged people to incorporate more plant-based options into their diets. Their status and influence in the culinary world enable them to reach a wide audience and inspire individuals to consider the impact of their food choices on their health and the environment. Celebrity chefs, through their cooking shows, cookbooks, and social media presence, have debunked the notion that plant-based diets are restrictive and unappealing while emphasizing the numerous health and environmental benefits associated with these diets. The promotion of plant-based diets by celebrity chefs has contributed to the growing acceptance and popularity of plant-based eating patterns in society.

PLANT-BASED DIETS AND FITNESS

Plant-based diets have gained popularity in recent years, not only for their environmental and ethical benefits but also for their potential impact on fitness and overall health. Many athletes and fitness enthusiasts are now adopting plant-based diets to enhance their performance and recovery. Research has shown that plant-based diets can provide ample amounts of essential nutrients, such as carbohydrates, protein, and fats, while also being low in saturated fats and cholesterol. Plant-based diets are rich in antioxidants, which can help reduce inflammation and oxidative stress caused by intense exercise. Plant-based diets are typically high in fiber, which aids in digestion and promotes satiety, leading to better weight management. Some studies have even suggested that plant-based diets may improve heart health, lower blood pressure, and reduce the risk of developing chronic diseases. It is important to note that athletes and individuals engaging in intense physical activity must ensure they consume sufficient calories and nutrients to meet their energy needs. Proper meal planning and consultation with a registered dietitian are crucial when transitioning to a plant-based diet to ensure optimal fitness and overall well-being.

PLANT-BASED NUTRITION FOR ATHLETES

Plant-based nutrition has gained significant popularity in recent years, and athletes are no exception to this trend. Contrary to the belief that athletes require animal proteins to meet their nutritional needs, research has shown that a well-planned plant-based diet can adequately support athletic performance. Plant-based diets are rich in complex carbohydrates, vitamins, minerals, fiber, and antioxidants that provide optimal fuel for physical activity and aid in muscle recovery. Plant-based proteins, such as those found in beans, legumes, and tofu, can provide the necessary amino acids for muscle growth and repair. Plant-based diets have been linked to a lower risk of chronic diseases and inflammation, which can be detrimental to an athlete's performance. Athletes who switch to plant-based nutrition often report improved energy levels, reduced post-exercise muscle soreness, and faster recovery times. While it is essential for athletes to carefully plan their plant-based diet to ensure adequate calorie and nutrient intake, the benefits of adopting a plant-based lifestyle for athletic performance cannot be overlooked.

RECOVERY AND PERFORMANCE BENEFITS

Athletes are constantly seeking ways to improve their performance and enhance their recovery after intense training and competitions. The plant-based revolution has provided them with a promising solution. Research studies have consistently shown that a diet rich in plant-based foods can have significant benefits in terms of recovery and performance. The high antioxidant content found in fruits and vegetables help reduce inflammation and oxidative stress inflicted by intense physical activity, improving the overall recovery process. Plant-based diets offer a rich source of carbohydrates, which are essential for replenishing glycogen stores in the muscles, ensuring optimal energy levels during workouts. Plant-based proteins, such as legumes and soy, are complete proteins and contain all essential amino acids required for muscle repair and growth. By incorporating more plant-based foods into their diet, athletes can promote faster recovery, reduce muscle soreness, enhance energy levels, and ultimately improve their performance on the field. With these benefits in mind, it is no surprise that an increasing number of athletes are embracing the plant-based revolution and reaping the rewards of a plant-powered lifestyle.

CASE STUDIES OF ATHLETES ON PLANT-BASED DIETS

have demonstrated the potential of this dietary approach to effectively fuel intensive physical activity. The case of Scott Jurek, an ultramarathoner and multiple-time winner of the Western States 100 Mile Endurance Run, showcases how a plant-based diet can support elite athletic performance. Jurek attributes his success and ability to recover quickly from grueling races to his plant-based lifestyle. Another noteworthy case is that of Patrik Baboumian, a world-record-holding strongman competitor. Baboumian has embraced a vegan diet to power his training and has achieved remarkable feats of strength, defying the misconception that animal products are necessary for building muscle mass. Venus Williams, one of the greatest tennis players of all time, has adopted a raw vegan diet in an effort to manage her auto-immune disease while maintaining a high level of performance on the court. These case studies highlight the potential benefits of plant-based diets for athletes in terms of improving endurance, recovery, and overall physical performance.

THE IMPACT ON ANIMAL POPULATIONS

As the plant-based revolution gains traction, its impact on animal populations cannot be overlooked.

With the increasing adoption of plant-based diets, there has been a visible shift in the demand for animal products, leading to a decline in the need for animal agriculture. This shift has undoubtedly contributed to the reduction of animal populations, particularly those bred for meat, dairy, and egg consumption. As a result, the strain on natural resources required to support the massive livestock industry has been curtailed. The decrease in animal agriculture has also led to a reduction in greenhouse gas emissions, water contamination, and deforestation associated with the industry. While the decline in animal populations may concern some who argue for the preservation of certain species, it is important to recognize the overall positive impact of this shift. The plant-based revolution provides an opportunity for a more sustainable relationship with animals, where their lives are not solely defined by human consumption. As individuals continue to embrace plant-based diets, the benefits for both the environment and animal populations will undoubtedly continue to grow.

REDUCTION IN LIVESTOCK NUMBERS

A reduction in livestock numbers is a crucial step towards achieving sustainability and addressing environmental concerns. Livestock production is a major contributor to greenhouse gas emissions, deforestation, and water pollution. By reducing the number of animals raised for food, we can significantly reduce our carbon footprint and mitigate the impacts of climate change. The amount of resources required for livestock farming is astronomical. Vast quantities of water, land, and feed are necessary to sustain the current demand for animal-based products. By transitioning to a plant-based diet, we can alleviate this strain on our natural resources and redirect them towards more sustainable practices. The reduction in livestock numbers would have a positive effect on human health. High intakes of animal products have been linked to an increased risk of several chronic diseases, including heart disease, diabetes, and certain cancers. Encouraging individuals to consume less meat and more plant-based foods can improve their overall health and well-being. A reduction in livestock numbers is not only beneficial for the environment but also for human health and the sustainable future of our planet.

WILDLIFE CONSERVATION EFFORTS

As the demand for animal products declines and vegan alternatives gain popularity, there is the potential for positive impacts on wildlife and biodiversity. The livestock industry is a major driver of deforestation and habitat loss, contributing to the decline of various species. By reducing the global consumption of animal products, we can alleviate the pressure on natural habitats and allow wildlife populations to recover. The shift towards plant-based diets can also lead to a decrease in hunting and poaching activities, which severely affect endangered animals. Wildlife conservation organizations are recognizing the potential of the plant-based revolution to mitigate the threats faced by numerous species. They advocate for sustainable agricultural practices and support the development of plant-based alternatives to animal products. These organizations raise awareness about the environmental consequences of the meat industry and its impact on wildlife. Through educational initiatives and public campaigns, they aim to foster a sense of responsibility and encourage individuals to make conscious choices that promote the well-being of both animals and their habitats.

THE RIPPLE EFFECT ON ECOSYSTEMS

The Plant-Based Revolution is not only impacting individuals and societies, but it is also creating a significant ripple effect on ecosystems. With the rise of plant-based diets, the demand for meat and animal products has decreased, leading to a decrease in the production of livestock. This decrease in livestock production has numerous positive effects on ecosystems. First, it reduces the amount of land needed for grazing and the associated deforestation. By minimizing deforestation, plant-based diets help preserve crucial habitats for countless species, ultimately contributing to biodiversity conservation. The reduction in livestock production also decreases the amount of water and energy required for their rearing. This reduction in resource consumption helps alleviate the strain on natural resources, benefiting ecosystems that rely on these resources for their survival. The decreased use of pesticides and fertilizers associated with raising animals for food also alleviates the pollution and detrimental impacts on ecosystems. Thus, the shift towards plant-based diets not only improves human health and well-being but also has far-reaching positive effects on ecosystems and the environment.

THE FUTURE OF FARMING WITH PLANT-BASED TRENDS

There has been a significant shift in consumer preferences towards plant-based diets, leading to the rise of the plant-based food industry. This trend has not only influenced the food market but also has the potential to reshape the future of farming. As demand for plant-based products continues to grow, farmers are expected to adapt and specialize in producing crops that cater to this new market. The shift to plant-based farming can have positive environmental implications, as it reduces the reliance on animal agriculture, which is a significant contributor to greenhouse gas emissions and deforestation. Plant-based farming requires less water and land compared to traditional livestock farming, making it a more sustainable and efficient option. To meet the increasing demand for plant-based foods, innovative technologies such as vertical farming and hydroponics can be implemented, ensuring year-round crop production and reducing the need for large expanses of agricultural land. As the plant-based revolution expands, farmers will need to embrace these trends and explore new ways to cultivate and optimize plant-based products, ultimately forging a greener and more sustainable future for farming.

SHIFTS IN AGRICULTURAL PRACTICES

A shift in agricultural practices is crucial for the plant-based revolution. Historically, traditional agricultural methods have relied heavily on intensive farming, leading to deforestation, soil erosion, and depletion of natural resources. The growing demand for plant-based foods has prompted a reevaluation of these practices. Sustainable farming practices such as organic farming, permaculture, and regenerative agriculture are gaining traction as viable alternatives. Organic farming emphasizes the use of natural fertilizers and pest control methods, reducing the reliance on synthetic inputs. Permaculture focuses on creating self-sustaining ecosystems, utilizing diverse plant species and animal interactions to enhance productivity and reduce waste. Regenerative agriculture aims to replenish and restore degraded soils through practices like cover cropping, crop rotation, and minimal tillage. These shifts in agricultural practices not only address environmental concerns but also improve the quality and nutritional value of plant-based foods. They contribute to a more sustainable and resilient food system that can support the growing global population without degrading the environment.

THE POTENTIAL FOR VERTICAL AND URBAN FARMING

One potential solution to the challenges of traditional agriculture is the concept of vertical and urban farming. Vertical farming refers to the practice of growing crops in vertically stacked layers, often in indoor environments. This approach maximizes the use of space and allows for year-round cultivation, regardless of weather conditions. Vertical farming can significantly reduce water usage by employing systems such as hydroponics or aeroponics, where plants are grown in nutrient-rich water solutions or in air with minimal water usage. Urban farming involves cultivating plants and raising animals within cities, utilizing both indoor and outdoor spaces. By bringing agriculture closer to urban centers, the distance between production and consumption is shortened, reducing carbon emissions associated with transportation. Urban farming also offers the possibility of producing local, fresh, and organic produce, decreasing the reliance on imported fruits and vegetables. These innovative farming methods can inspire local communities to actively participate in local food production, fostering a sense of connection to the environment and promoting sustainable practices. Vertical and urban farming have the potential to revolutionize how we produce food, making it more accessible, environmentally-friendly, and resilient to external factors.

THE ROLE OF TECHNOLOGY IN PLANT-BASED AGRICULTURE

With the growing demand for sustainable and cruelty-free food options, technology has played a vital role in enhancing productivity, efficiency, and innovation in plant-based agriculture. One notable technology that has revolutionized the industry is vertical farming. By utilizing stackable trays or shelves with hydroponic systems, vertical farms enable food production in limited spaces with controlled environments, eliminating the need for large areas of land and reducing water usage. Advanced greenhouse technologies have allowed for year-round cultivation of crops, making it easier to meet the increasing demand for plant-based products. Biotechnology and genetic engineering techniques have been pivotal in the development of genetically modified crops that exhibit desirable traits such as increased yields or resistance to pests and diseases. These technological advancements not only ensure the availability of high-quality plant-based products but also contribute to the overall sustainability and environmental friendliness of the agriculture industry in the face of global challenges such as climate change and food scarcity.

THE ROLE OF EDUCATION IN THE PLANT-BASED REVOLUTION

Education plays a pivotal role in the plant-based revolution, as it has the potential to drive the necessary behavioral changes in individuals towards adopting a plant-based lifestyle. By providing individuals with accurate information about the health benefits, ethical concerns, and environmental impact of consuming animal products, education can empower them to make informed choices. A key aspect of this educational approach is promoting the understanding of the interconnections between personal health, the well-being of animals, and the sustainability of the planet. This type of education can be integrated into various levels of the education system, ranging from primary education to higher education. Schools can incorporate plant-based nutrition education into their curricula, ensuring that young students are exposed to the benefits of a plant-based diet from an early age. Colleges and universities can offer courses, workshops, and seminars on plant-based nutrition, highlighting the scientific evidence supporting its benefits. In addition to formal education, public awareness campaigns and initiatives can also play a vital role in disseminating information and fostering a culture of plant-based living. Education serves as a crucial catalyst for the plant-based revolution by equipping individuals with the knowledge necessary to make healthier and more sustainable choices.

CURRICULUM CHANGES IN SCHOOLS AND UNIVERSITIES

As society becomes increasingly aware of the negative impacts of traditional eating habits, educational institutions have realized the need to adapt their curricula to reflect this paradigm shift. This transformation involves incorporating comprehensive and balanced nutrition education that emphasizes the benefits of a plant-based diet. By doing so, schools and universities can equip students with the knowledge and skills needed to make informed dietary choices, contributing to their overall health and well-being. Curriculum changes encompass a broader perspective, integrating the study of sustainability and environmental issues associated with animal agriculture. Students are exposed to the ecological consequences of intensive farming practices, as well as the potential of plant-based diets to mitigate these concerns. By incorporating these topics into the educational system, schools and universities are not only addressing the immediate health needs of students, but also paving the way for a more sustainable and compassionate future. As the plant-based revolution gains momentum, it is crucial for educational institutions to recognize their role in preparing the next generation to embrace and promote healthier dietary choices.

PUBLIC WORKSHOPS AND COOKING CLASSES

These educational opportunities provide a platform to learn about the benefits of plant-based diets and gain practical skills in preparing nutritious and delicious meals. Often led by experienced chefs or nutrition experts, these workshops offer a structured setting for participants to ask questions, acquire information, and receive hands-on guidance. Through interactive demonstrations and tasting sessions, attendees can explore a variety of plant-based ingredients, cooking techniques, and recipe ideas. Public workshops and cooking classes also promote community engagement and networking, allowing attendees to connect with like-minded individuals who share similar dietary goals and interests. These forums provide a safe space for individuals to discuss challenges or seek advice from experts and peers. By equipping participants with the knowledge and skills needed to navigate the plant-based world, public workshops and cooking classes play a vital role in empowering individuals to embrace a healthier, more sustainable diet.

ONLINE RESOURCES AND EDUCATIONAL PLATFORMS

With the rise of technology, individuals now have access to a wealth of information related to plant-based diets and sustainable living. Online platforms such as websites, blogs, and social media have become valuable sources of knowledge, providing a wide range of recipes, nutritional information, and lifestyle tips. Educational platforms like online courses and webinars have emerged, offering comprehensive and in-depth learning experiences. These resources not only educate individuals on the health benefits of plant-based diets but also highlight the environmental and ethical advantages of adopting a plant-based lifestyle. Online communities and forums have also played a pivotal role in connecting like-minded individuals, fostering a sense of support and inspiration. The accessibility and convenience of online resources have allowed people from diverse backgrounds and geographical locations to participate in the plant-based movement. Online resources and educational platforms have revolutionized the way information is shared and accessed, empowering individuals to embrace a plant-based lifestyle and contribute to a more sustainable future.

THE INFLUENCE OF RELIGION AND SPIRITUALITY

Religion and spirituality have long played a significant role in shaping human beliefs, values, and behaviors. These two interconnected dimensions have shaped not only personal lives but also societies and cultures throughout history. The influence of religion and spirituality transcends the boundaries of individual faiths, touching various aspects of life including ethics, social interactions, and even dietary choices. The influence of religion can be particularly apparent in dietary practices, as many religious traditions prescribe specific dietary restrictions and guidelines. Followers of Judaism adhere to kosher dietary laws, abstaining from the consumption of certain foods such as pork and shellfish. Similarly, Hinduism and Buddhism advocate for vegetarianism as a means of practicing compassion and non-violence towards all living beings. Many religions and spiritual practices emphasize mindfulness and the importance of being present in the moment, which can greatly impact individuals' approach to food and eating. The influence of religion and spirituality on dietary choices demonstrates the integral role that these dimensions play in shaping human behaviors, including the choices we make regarding our food consumption.

RELIGIOUS DOCTRINES ADVOCATING FOR PLANT-BASED EATING

In recent decades, there has been a significant increase in the number of individuals embracing plant-based diets, driven by various motivations including health concerns and environmental sustainability. Interestingly, religious doctrines have also played a part in advocating for plant-based eating. Some religious traditions emphasize the sanctity of life and promote the idea of reducing harm to sentient beings. In Hinduism, followers are encouraged to adopt a vegetarian or vegan lifestyle as a means of practicing ahimsa, or non-violence. Similarly, Jainism advocates for vegetarianism as a way to uphold the principle of ahimsa and avoid causing harm to any living being. Buddhism also guides its followers towards a plant-based diet through its teachings on compassion and avoiding harm. In certain Christian denominations, fasting or abstaining from animal products is observed during specific religious periods, such as Lent. These religious doctrines not only promote a more compassionate and ethical approach to food choices, but also align with the growing scientific evidence supporting the health benefits of plant-based diets. As a result, individuals who adhere to these religious beliefs find themselves aligning with the plant-based revolution, thus contributing to its momentum.

SPIRITUAL PERSPECTIVES ON NON-VIOLENCE AND DIET

Various religious and spiritual traditions emphasize the importance of non-violence and compassion towards all living beings. Hinduism promotes Ahimsa, the principle of non-harm, and encourages the consumption of a vegetarian diet to minimize harm to animals. Similarly, Buddhism emphasizes the concept of interconnectedness and the idea that all sentient beings are interconnected in a vast web of life. This notion informs Buddhist practitioners to adopt a diet that respects and minimizes the suffering of all living beings. Jainism advocates for the principle of Ahimsa at its core, prescribing a diet that avoids violence towards any living being, including plants. These spiritual perspectives acknowledge the interconnectedness of all life forms and emphasize the ethical and moral responsibility towards all sentient beings. By adopting a plant-based diet, individuals align themselves with these spiritual beliefs, recognizing the importance of non-violence and compassion towards both humans and animals. Thus, spirituality plays a crucial role in promoting the adoption of a plant-based lifestyle, as it provides a strong moral foundation and ethical framework for making dietary choices.

RELIGIOUS COMMUNITIES AND PLANT-BASED INITIATIVES

Religious communities have begun to embrace plant-based initiatives as a way to align their beliefs with their dietary choices. Many religious doctrines promote the idea of compassion towards animals and the environment, making plant-based living an attractive option for their followers. Jainism, a religion that originated in ancient India, emphasizes non-violence and non-possession, promoting a vegan lifestyle as a means to avoid harm to all living beings. Similarly, Buddhism encourages its adherents to practice mindfulness and compassion, and many Buddhists choose to adopt a plant-based diet for ethical reasons. Some Christian denominations have also started to emphasize the importance of sustainable and ethical food choices, urging their followers to consider the environmental impact of animal agriculture and support plant-based alternatives. Religious communities often have a strong sense of community and collective values, making them effective catalysts for change. By embracing plant-based initiatives, religious communities can not only align their dietary choices with their beliefs but also inspire their followers to make more conscious and compassionate choices in their daily lives.

LEGAL AND REGULATORY ASPECTS

As the plant-based revolution gains momentum, it is crucial to consider the legal and regulatory aspects surrounding this novel industry. Various legal frameworks, such as intellectual property laws, are becoming critical to protect the innovations and investments made in the plant-based sector. Companies involved in developing and scaling up plant-based products face the challenge of securing patents and trademarks for their unique technologies and product formulations. Regulations concerning labeling and marketing claims for plant-based products need to be established to ensure consumer transparency and fair competition with traditional animal-based products. This is particularly important as the plant-based industry continues to expand and more products enter the market. Government agencies and policymakers must address the need for standardized definitions and regulations regarding terms like "vegan," "vegetarian," and "plant-based" to prevent confusion and misleading statements. With proper legal and regulatory frameworks in place, the plant-based revolution can flourish, bringing about a healthier and more sustainable future for both human health and the environment.

LABELING LAWS FOR PLANT-BASED PRODUCTS

With more consumers opting for plant-based alternatives to meat and dairy products, the need for accurate and transparent labeling has become paramount. One issue that arises is the use of terms like "milk" or "cheese" to describe plant-based products. Some argue that these terms should be reserved exclusively for animal-derived products, as their use in plant-based goods can mislead consumers. On the other hand, proponents of plant-based products argue that these terms can help consumers understand the purpose and use of the products more easily. Labeling laws can address concerns related to allergies by clearly indicating the presence of common allergens in plant-based products. Accurate labeling can help consumers make informed choices about their dietary preferences and can contribute to the overall growth and acceptance of the plant-based market. As the plant-based revolution continues to gain momentum, it is crucial to establish clear and comprehensive labeling requirements to ensure consumer protection and promote transparency within the industry.

REGULATIONS ON PLANT-BASED FOOD PRODUCTION

As the demand for plant-based alternatives increases, it becomes imperative to establish regulations that protect consumer health and prevent fraudulent practices. In the United States, the Food and Drug Administration (FDA) plays a significant role in regulating plant-based food production. The FDA mandates strict guidelines for labeling and ingredients declaration, ensuring transparency and preventing misrepresentation. Regulations cover aspects such as manufacturing practices and allergen control, guaranteeing that plant-based products meet stringent safety standards. These regulations are crucial to assure consumers that plant-based food products are produced under sanitary conditions and are free from any harmful contaminants. Regulations also serve to maintain fair competition in the market, preventing deceptive claims and ensuring a level playing field among producers. By enforcing these regulations, consumers can have confidence in the safety and integrity of the plant-based food they consume, fostering the continued growth and acceptance of plant-based options as a reliable and healthy alternative to traditional animal-derived products.

LEGAL CHALLENGES FACED BY THE PLANT-BASED INDUSTRY

One key challenge involves the labeling of plant-based products, particularly those that aim to imitate traditionally animal-based foods. Some regulatory bodies require plant-based foods to have specific labeling that identifies them as plant-based, while others argue that such labeling may confuse consumers. This legal debate raises questions about transparency and consumer understanding. Another legal challenge revolves around intellectual property rights, particularly in relation to plant-based meat substitutes. Companies in the plant-based industry are developing new technologies and processes to create meat substitutes that resemble animal meat in taste and texture. This has led to legal disputes and claims of intellectual property infringement. The plant-based industry faces regulatory challenges regarding food safety, nutritional claims, and compositional standards. As the industry continues to grow and innovate, it will be important to navigate these legal complexities to ensure consumer trust and a level playing field for plant-based businesses.

THE PSYCHOLOGY OF CHANGE AND DIETARY SHIFTS

The psychology of change plays a crucial role in understanding the adoption of dietary shifts, particularly when it comes to embracing a plant-based lifestyle. This transformation involves not only a change in eating habits but also a shift from a long-held cultural and societal norm. In examining the psychology behind this change, several factors come to light. First and foremost, individuals must overcome the resistance to change, which stems from fear of the unknown and a discomfort with breaking away from established routines and traditions. The psychology of change acknowledges that humans tend to be creatures of habit, finding comfort in familiarity. When individuals consider shifting towards a plant-based diet, they must confront the challenge of breaking these deeply ingrained habits and beliefs. Psychological research reveals that change is more likely to occur when individuals experience a personal connection or identify with a cause. Understanding the values and motivations that drive people to switch to a plant-based lifestyle becomes pivotal in influencing dietary shifts. By understanding the psychological processes involved, researchers and advocates can employ strategic approaches to facilitate and support individuals in successfully transitioning to a plant-based diet.

STAGES OF BEHAVIORAL CHANGE IN DIET MODIFICATION

One of the key factors in successful diet modification is understanding the stages of behavioral change. According to the Transtheoretical Model, there are six stages individuals go through when attempting to change their eating habits. The first stage is precontemplation, where individuals have no intention of altering their diet. This is followed by contemplation, where people start to acknowledge the need for change and consider different options. The third stage is preparation, where individuals start to plan and gather tools necessary for the diet modification. Action is the next stage, where individuals actually begin implementing the changes into their daily lives. Maintenance, the fifth stage, refers to the long-term practice of the modified diet. The sixth stage is termination, where the modified diet becomes ingrained and individuals no longer have the desire or need to revert to their old eating habits. Understanding these stages can help individuals navigate the process of diet modification and anticipate the challenges and successes that may arise. By recognizing where one is in the process, individuals can tailor their approach and increase their chances of long-term success in adopting a plant-based diet.

STRATEGIES FOR SUCCESSFUL TRANSITION TO PLANT-BASED EATING

Strategies for a successful transition to plant-based eating require careful planning, education, and dedication. First and foremost, individuals should draw up a detailed meal plan that includes a variety of fruits, vegetables, legumes, whole grains, and plant-based proteins. This not only ensures a well-balanced diet but also helps in successfully substituting animal-based products. Learning about plant-based nutrition is equally important, as it helps individuals understand the nutrient composition of various plant-based foods and ensures that they meet their daily nutritional requirements. It is essential to gradually transition to a plant-based diet rather than adopting it abruptly, as sudden changes may lead to discomfort and potential nutrient deficiencies. By slowly incorporating plant-based meals into their diet and gradually reducing animal-based products, individuals can adjust their taste preferences, digestion, and overall well-being. Seeking support from communities, such as plant-based eating groups or online forums, can provide a sense of community and offer valuable insights and advice. Successful transition to plant-based eating requires commitment, patience, and a willingness to experiment with new flavors and ingredients.

OVERCOMING PSYCHOLOGICAL BARRIERS

Many individuals have deeply ingrained beliefs and habits that revolve around the consumption of animal products, making it difficult for them to even consider a plant-based diet. The psychological barriers that prevent people from making this shift stem from a variety of sources, including cultural norms, family traditions, and personal taste preferences. There is a fear of missing out on certain nutrients and a concern about social implications, which can contribute to the resistance towards change. To overcome these barriers, individuals need to challenge their preconceived notions and open themselves up to new possibilities. Education plays a significant role in this process, as it provides a deeper understanding of the benefits of a plant-based lifestyle and dispels myths surrounding nutritional adequacy. Creating a supportive network of like-minded individuals can provide the necessary encouragement and motivation. By gradually introducing plant-based alternatives into their diets and exploring new recipes and flavors, individuals can gradually overcome their psychological barriers and embrace the plant-based revolution.

THE ROLE OF NON-PROFIT ORGANIZATIONS

Non-profit organizations play a crucial role in advancing the plant-based revolution. These organizations provide essential support in promoting plant-based diets, environmental conservation, and animal rights. Through their advocacy efforts, non-profit organizations raise awareness about the negative impacts of animal agriculture on our planet and encourage individuals to adopt plant-based lifestyles as a solution. These organizations often conduct scientific research to identify the health benefits of plant-based diets and share this information with the public. By organizing public campaigns and events, they effectively reach a wide audience, encouraging individuals to make conscious choices that align with their values. Non-profit organizations often collaborate with educational institutions, government agencies, and businesses to develop and implement initiatives that promote plant-based diets at a larger scale. They also focus on lobbying for policy changes that support sustainable farming practices and stricter regulations for the meat industry. By driving innovation in the food industry and supporting communities through education and resources, non-profit organizations are instrumental in transforming our society into one that prioritizes sustainable, ethical, and plant-based practices.

ADVOCACY AND AWARENESS CAMPAIGNS

These campaigns aim to educate the public about the health benefits of consuming plant-based foods while highlighting the negative consequences of a meat-centric diet. By doing so, they raise awareness about the impact of animal agriculture on the environment, animal welfare, and human health. Advocacy campaigns often involve collaborating with influential figures, celebrities, and experts who can lend credibility to the cause and attract attention from a wider audience. Social media platforms have become powerful tools for disseminating information and engaging with individuals on a global scale. With the increasing popularity of plant-based diets, advocacy campaigns have the potential to shift societal norms and cultural perceptions surrounding food choices. By emphasizing the positive aspects of embracing a plant-based lifestyle, such as improved health, a reduced carbon footprint, and reduced animal suffering, these campaigns have the power to inspire individuals to make more conscious and compassionate choices about what they eat.

SUPPORT NETWORKS FOR PLANT-BASED COMMUNITIES

Support networks play a crucial role in the success and growth of plant-based communities. These communities are formed by individuals who choose to adopt a plant-based lifestyle, either for health, environmental, or ethical reasons. Support networks provide a sense of community and belonging, as well as offering resources, information, and encouragement to those who are transitioning to or maintaining a plant-based diet. Online platforms, such as social media groups, forums, and websites dedicated to plant-based living, have emerged as valuable support networks. These platforms allow individuals to connect with like-minded individuals, share their experiences, seek advice, and find inspiration. Plant-based communities also organize offline events and gatherings, such as cooking workshops, potlucks, and educational talks, which provide individuals with the opportunity to meet others face-to-face and build relationships. These support networks not only facilitate the sharing of knowledge and experiences but also serve as a source of motivation, encouragement, and accountability. Support networks are essential in creating a supportive and empowering environment for plant-based individuals, enabling them to thrive and continue on their journey towards a more sustainable and compassionate lifestyle.

RESEARCH FUNDING AND DISSEMINATION

As the plant-based movement gains momentum, it is necessary to secure funding for research in order to understand the benefits and potential drawbacks of this dietary shift. Research funding is essential for conducting studies that can provide evidence-based support for the health benefits of plant-based diets, as well as investigate the environmental and ethical implications of animal agriculture. The dissemination of research findings plays a vital role in communicating the benefits of plant-based diets to the wider public and encouraging behavior change. This can be achieved through academic publications, conferences, and public lectures. Investing in the development and promotion of easily accessible resources, such as online databases and educational materials, can increase the visibility and availability of research findings. By prioritizing research funding and dissemination, society can ensure that accurate information about the benefits of adopting a plant-based diet is readily available to individuals, communities, and policymakers, ultimately facilitating the plant-based revolution.

THE IMPACT ON THE HEALTHCARE SYSTEM

The rise of the plant-based revolution is having a profound impact on the healthcare system. As more people adopt a plant-based diet, there has been a significant decrease in chronic diseases such as cardiovascular disease, obesity, and diabetes. Several studies have shown that a diet rich in fruits, vegetables, whole grains, and legumes can help lower blood pressure, reduce cholesterol levels, and improve overall heart health. With these positive outcomes, the demand for expensive medical treatments and medications for chronic conditions has decreased, resulting in substantial cost savings for individuals and the healthcare system as a whole. The increased consumption of plant-based foods has also led to a reduction in the environmental impact associated with animal agriculture, such as deforestation, greenhouse gas emissions, and water pollution. These environmental benefits further contribute to the overall sustainability of the healthcare system by mitigating the negative consequences of industrial farming practices. The plant-based revolution is reshaping the healthcare system by promoting healthier lifestyles, reducing disease prevalence, and improving both individual and environmental well-being.

POTENTIAL FOR REDUCED HEALTHCARE COSTS

One significant potential benefit of a plant-based diet is the potential for reduced healthcare costs. Chronic diseases such as obesity, diabetes, and heart disease are prevalent in society, often resulting in substantial healthcare expenditures. Research has indicated that a plant-based diet can contribute to the prevention and management of these illnesses. Studies have shown that individuals who follow a plant-based diet have a lower risk of developing type 2 diabetes compared to those who consume a typical Western diet. This is primarily due to the higher intake of fiber, antioxidants, and phytochemicals found in plant-based foods, which help regulate blood sugar levels and improve insulin sensitivity. Plant-based diets have been associated with lower blood pressure and cholesterol levels, reducing the risk of developing cardiovascular diseases. By adopting a plant-based diet, individuals may experience a decrease in healthcare costs related to medications, hospitalizations, and treatments for chronic diseases. Thus, promoting a plant-based revolution in dietary patterns can potentially alleviate the burden on healthcare systems, contributing to overall cost reductions in healthcare expenditures.

PLANT-BASED DIETS IN CLINICAL SETTINGS

Plant-based diets have gained popularity in recent years due to their numerous health benefits. In clinical settings, these diets have been shown to have positive effects on various chronic diseases. Research has shown that adopting a plant-based diet can help manage diabetes by improving blood sugar control and reducing the need for medication. Plant-based diets have been associated with a lower risk of developing heart disease and high blood pressure. This is primarily attributed to their high fiber content, which helps lower cholesterol levels and maintain a healthy weight. Plant-based diets have also shown promise in the prevention and management of certain types of cancer. Studies have found that individuals who consume a predominantly plant-based diet have a reduced risk of developing prostate, breast, and colon cancer. Plant-based diets can also alleviate symptoms and improve outcomes in patients with certain autoimmune diseases, such as rheumatoid arthritis. Incorporating plant-based diets into clinical settings can be a valuable and effective strategy for improving patient outcomes and promoting healthier lifestyles.

TRAINING HEALTHCARE PROFESSIONALS ON PLANT-BASED NUTRITION

Although the benefits of plant-based diets have been widely recognized, many healthcare professionals receive minimal education on nutrition during their training, with even fewer resources dedicated to plant-based nutrition specifically. This knowledge gap can hinder their ability to offer evidence-based guidance to patients seeking to adopt a plant-based diet. By equipping healthcare professionals with the necessary training on plant-based nutrition, they can better understand the appropriate nutrient composition and potential deficiencies associated with this dietary approach. They can effectively address concerns and provide tailored advice to individuals considering plant-based diets for health reasons or ethical considerations. This training should cover topics such as the essential nutrients provided by plants, meal planning, potential food substitutions, and strategies for ensuring adequate nutrient intake. By incorporating plant-based nutrition education into medical and healthcare curricula, healthcare professionals can play a pivotal role in promoting plant-based diets as a viable and sustainable solution for improving both individual and public health.

THE ROLE OF TECHNOLOGY IN THE PLANT-BASED REVOLUTION

In the plant-based revolution, technology plays a crucial role in enabling the development and widespread adoption of plant-based products. Advances in biotechnology have allowed for the engineering of plant-based alternatives that closely mimic the taste, texture, and nutritional profile of animal-based products. Through techniques such as genetic modification and cellular agriculture, scientists are able to create plant-based proteins that meet the demands of consumers seeking sustainable and ethical food choices. Technological innovations have also made it possible to scale up the production of plant-based foods, making them more accessible and affordable for the masses. From precision farming methods to automated food processing, technology has revolutionized the plant-based industry, ensuring a steady supply of high-quality products. Technology has also played a significant role in promoting the plant-based movement through social media platforms, online communities, and recipe-sharing apps. These digital platforms have facilitated knowledge-sharing, connected like-minded individuals, and amplified the reach of plant-based advocates. Without technology, the plant-based revolution would not have gained the momentum and global impact we see today.

APPS AND TOOLS FOR PLANT-BASED LIVING

One of the most prominent ways in which technology is supporting the plant-based revolution is through the development of various apps and tools that cater specifically to the needs of those living a plant-based lifestyle. These innovative applications provide users with a wide range of resources to aid in their pursuit of plant-based living. There are apps available that offer recipe suggestions and meal planning features, allowing individuals to effortlessly incorporate plant-based meals into their daily routine. Some apps provide comprehensive nutritional information and guidance, ensuring that users are meeting their dietary requirements while adhering to a plant-based diet. There are tools that allow individuals to track their plant-based journey, monitor their progress, and connect with like-minded individuals through social networking features. These apps and tools have become invaluable companions for those embracing a plant-based lifestyle, providing them with the necessary support and resources to navigate their journey with ease and confidence.

THE DEVELOPMENT OF LAB-GROWN MEAT

Lab-grown meat, also known as cultured meat or cell-based meat, refers to the production of meat products using tissue engineering techniques instead of traditional livestock farming. This innovative approach offers several benefits that address the environmental, ethical, and health concerns associated with conventional meat production. Firstly, lab-grown meat has the potential to reduce the greenhouse gas emissions generated by livestock farming. By cultivating meat directly from animal cells in controlled lab environments, it eliminates the need for extensive land use, deforestation, and methane emissions associated with livestock. This technology presents a more humane approach to meat production as it does not involve the slaughter of animals. It also eliminates the risk of foodborne illnesses and the need for antibiotics commonly used in traditional meat production. Lab-grown meat has the potential to provide a more sustainable and resource-efficient solution to feed the growing global population. By revolutionizing the way we produce meat, lab-grown meat has the power to reshape the future of the food industry.

TECHNOLOGY'S ROLE IN PLANT-BASED FOOD DISTRIBUTION

Technology plays a crucial role in the distribution of plant-based food products. As the demand for plant-based alternatives continues to rise, advancements in technology have facilitated the effective distribution of these products to consumers across the globe. One important aspect of technology in plant-based food distribution is the development of sustainable packaging solutions. Companies have been able to use biodegradable and compostable materials for packaging, reducing the environmental impact of the distribution process. Technology has enabled the creation of innovative transportation systems, ensuring that plant-based products are delivered efficiently and in a timely manner. With the help of tracking technologies, companies can monitor the movement of goods, ensuring freshness and quality during transportation. Technology has played a pivotal role in the establishment of e-commerce platforms for plant-based products, making them easily accessible to consumers. These online platforms use advanced algorithms to recommend products tailored to individual preferences, making the purchasing experience seamless and convenient. Technology has significantly contributed to the growth and accessibility of plant-based food distribution, promoting sustainable choices and a healthier lifestyle.

THE INTERSECTION OF PLANT-BASED DIETS AND POLITICS

The rise of plant-based diets has given birth to a socio-political movement that aims to challenge the status quo of conventional food systems. The increasing popularity of plant-based diets is not simply a matter of personal health choices, but rather a conscientious effort to address larger issues such as sustainability, animal rights, and climate change. At the intersection of plant-based diets and politics, individuals and organizations have begun advocating for legislative and policy changes that support the growth and accessibility of plant-based food options. This movement recognizes that dietary choices have far-reaching implications on the environment, public health, and society at large. By promoting dietary changes that rely less on animal products and more on plant-based alternatives, proponents of this movement are pushing for a reevaluation of governmental policies related to food production, subsidies, and labeling. They aim to influence education and public awareness campaigns to illuminate the benefits of plant-based diets and encourage a shift away from conventional meat-centered diets. As plant-based diets gain traction, the political landscape must adapt to accommodate the changing demands of an increasingly eco-conscious population.

POLITICAL ADVOCACY FOR PLANT-BASED POLICIES

Advocates argue that promoting and implementing plant-based policies can address multiple crises simultaneously, including climate change, deforestation, and resource depletion. One of the key strategies used by proponents of plant-based policies is lobbying for government support and regulation to incentivize a shift towards plant-based diets and agriculture. They argue that governments need to provide financial incentives, such as subsidies and tax breaks, to promote the production and consumption of plant-based foods, while also implementing regulations that restrict the expansion of industrial animal agriculture. Supporters of plant-based policies also emphasize the health benefits of promoting plant-based diets, including reduced risk of chronic diseases like obesity, diabetes, and heart disease. They argue that political advocacy for plant-based policies can not only improve environmental sustainability but also enhance public health and well-being. Opponents raise concerns about potential job losses in the animal agriculture sector and challenges associated with dietary change on a large scale. Despite these concerns, the momentum behind political advocacy for plant-based policies continues to grow, with many governments starting to recognize the urgency and benefits of transitioning towards more plant-based systems.

THE INFLUENCE OF LOBBYISTS AND INTEREST GROUPS

Lobbyists, representing various industries, employ persuasive tactics to sway lawmakers in favor of their own interests. In the case of plant-based foods, interest groups such as those representing major agriculture corporations and animal welfare organizations exert considerable pressure to advance their respective agendas. Agriculture lobbyists may seek to block regulations or subsidies that promote plant-based alternatives, fearing potential economic impacts on traditional livestock farming sectors. Conversely, animal welfare groups strive to secure tighter regulations on animal agriculture practices, advocating for plant-based alternatives as a more ethical and sustainable solution. The tussle between these competing interest groups influences not only policy decisions but also public discourse surrounding plant-based foods. Lobbyists and interest groups leverage campaign contributions and other financial incentives to gain political support, further amplifying their influence. Consequently, the influence exerted by these actors necessitates a comprehensive understanding of their motivations and the potential biases they may introduce in shaping the plant-based revolution.

PLANT-BASED DIETS IN POLITICAL DISCOURSE

Plant-based diets have gained increasing attention and significance within political discourse. The intersections between diet, health, and the environment have brought plant-based diets to the forefront of political discussions. Policymakers and elected officials are now considering the incorporation of plant-based diets into governmental initiatives as a means to tackle both the obesity epidemic and climate change. Recognition of the detrimental effects of animal agriculture on greenhouse gas emissions has led to calls for the promotion of plant-based diets as a sustainable and eco-friendly solution. The growing awareness of the health benefits associated with plant-based diets has prompted political figures to advocate for their inclusion in public health programs. The adoption of plant-based diets as a political issue is not without controversy. Criticisms include concerns over the deprivation of traditional food culture and the potential negative impacts on farmers and the agricultural industry. Nonetheless, the inclusion of plant-based diets in political discourse highlights their growing influence and the urgent need to address the complex relationship between food, environment, and health through legislative means.

THE MEDIA'S ROLE IN SHAPING PERCEPTIONS

The media plays a significant role in shaping and influencing public perceptions. In the context of the plant-based revolution, the media has a pivotal role in disseminating information to the masses and consequently altering societal attitudes towards a plant-based lifestyle. Through various platforms, such as television, newspapers, and social media, the media provides a platform for experts, celebrities, and influencers to express their opinions, thus shaping public discourse. The media's power lies in its ability to frame issues and mold public opinion. By highlighting the environmental benefits of a plant-based diet or showcasing the success stories of individuals who have adopted this lifestyle, the media can reinforce positive perceptions and create a sense of desirability around plant-based living. It is important to note that media outlets are not immune to biases or influences from external factors. It is crucial for consumers to critically analyze the information presented by the media, considering different perspectives and sources. The media possesses a formidable power to shape and alter perceptions, making it a crucial player in the plant-based revolution.

COVERAGE OF PLANT-BASED DIETS IN NEWS OUTLETS

Another important aspect of the plant-based revolution is the coverage it receives in news outlets. With the increasing popularity and acceptance of plant-based diets, news outlets have devoted more attention to this topic in recent years. This coverage plays a crucial role in spreading awareness and providing information to the general public about the benefits and challenges of adopting a plant-based lifestyle. Many news outlets have published articles and featured segments on television shows that discuss the health benefits, environmental impact, and ethical considerations of plant-based diets. They have often interviewed experts in the field, including nutritionists, doctors, and researchers, to provide a comprehensive understanding of the subject matter. It is important to note that not all news outlets provide unbiased coverage. Some may be influenced by the interests of certain industries or have a tendency to sensationalize certain aspects of the plant-based movement. It is imperative for readers and viewers to critically evaluate the sources of information and seek multiple perspectives to form a well-rounded understanding of plant-based diets.

DOCUMENTARIES AND FILMS PROMOTING PLANT-BASED LIVING

By presenting compelling narratives and evidence-based arguments, these works have educated and inspired audiences to reconsider their dietary choices and embrace a plant-based diet. One such documentary is "Cowspiracy: The Sustainability Secret," which exposes the environmental impact of animal agriculture and argues for the adoption of plant-based eating as a means to mitigate climate change. Another notable film is "Forks Over Knives," which examines the health benefits of a plant-based diet and presents compelling evidence linking animal products to chronic diseases. By harnessing the power of visual storytelling, these documentaries not only educate viewers about the interconnectedness of our food choices and their consequences but also empower individuals to take action and make informed decisions about their diets. These films have also contributed to the normalization of plant-based living, debunking common misconceptions and highlighting the delicious variety and accessibility of plant-based foods. With their ability to reach diverse audiences, documentaries and films promoting plant-based living are pivotal in catalyzing the plant-based revolution and fostering a more sustainable and compassionate world.

THE PORTRAYAL OF PLANT-BASED DIETS IN POPULAR CULTURE

Traditionally, plant-based diets were often seen as niche or even extreme, associated with hippies or health fanatics. With the rise of social media and the increasing awareness of the environmental and health benefits of plant-based eating, these diets have gained mainstream popularity. Popular culture has played a crucial role in this transformation, as celebrities and influencers have become vocal advocates for plant-based lifestyles, sharing their personal experiences and promoting vegan and vegetarian options. Popular documentaries like "Forks Over Knives" and "Cowspiracy" have shed light on the detrimental effects of animal agriculture on the planet, further fueling the conversation around plant-based diets. The food industry has responded to this growing demand, with an array of plant-based alternatives, from burgers to dairy-free milk, becoming more accessible in supermarkets and restaurants. As a result, plant-based eating is becoming increasingly normalized and embraced as a trendy and ethical choice. Nevertheless, the portrayal of plant-based diets in popular culture can sometimes oversimplify the complexity of dietary choices and fail to recognize potential nutritional challenges for individuals.

THE ECONOMICS OF PLANT-BASED FOOD PRODUCTION

The global shift towards plant-based diets has not only been driven by concerns for personal health and environmental sustainability, but also by economic factors. The economics of plant-based food production offer a compelling argument for adopting a more plant-focused approach to our diets. Plants require fewer resources and emit fewer greenhouse gases compared to traditional animal agriculture. As a result, the production of plant-based foods is often more cost-effective and less environmentally damaging. The increasing demand for plant-based products has sparked innovation in the food industry, leading to new businesses and job opportunities. The growth of the plant-based market has also attracted investments from venture capitalists and institutions, driving the expansion of the industry and creating a positive feedback loop. Plant-based alternatives to animal products have become more affordable and accessible, making it easier for consumers to adopt a healthier and more sustainable lifestyle. Consequently, the economics of plant-based food production highlight the potential for a transformative shift in the global food system, benefiting both individual consumers and the planet as a whole.

COST ANALYSIS OF PLANT-BASED FOOD MANUFACTURING

A cost analysis of plant-based food manufacturing is crucial in understanding the viability and sustainability of this emerging industry. It is evident that the increasing popularity of plant-based diets and the long-term environmental consequences of animal agriculture necessitate a comprehensive examination of the economic aspects associated with plant-based food production. Costs incurred in plant-based food manufacturing include raw materials, labor, overhead, and marketing. Raw materials, such as fruits, vegetables, grains, and legumes, are typically cheaper and more abundant compared to animal-based ingredients. Labor costs can be lower in plant-based food manufacturing due to the decreased complexity and handling required in processing plant-based ingredients. Overhead costs, including energy consumption and machinery maintenance, can be reduced by utilizing energy-efficient technologies and sustainable practices. Marketing costs may pose a potential challenge for plant-based food manufacturers, as this industry is still relatively niche compared to the mainstream meat and dairy markets. A detailed cost analysis of plant-based food manufacturing will provide valuable insights into the economic feasibility and potential profitability of this industry while considering the associated environmental benefits.

ECONOMIC INCENTIVES FOR PLANT-BASED BUSINESSES

Economic incentives play a crucial role in encouraging the growth and development of plant-based businesses. Firstly, government subsidies can alleviate the financial burden on these businesses, making it easier for them to compete with traditional meat-based industries. By providing financial support in the form of grants and tax incentives, governments can incentivize the adoption of plant-based practices, allowing businesses to invest in research and development, expand production capabilities, and reduce costs. Policies promoting plant-based diets can also help stimulate consumer demand for plant-based products. Tax breaks for individuals who follow a plant-based diet or financial incentives for institutions that offer plant-based options in their menus can encourage more people to opt for these alternatives. Some countries have introduced carbon pricing mechanisms, which aim to address the environmental impact of food production. This puts plant-based businesses at an advantage as their production processes typically have lower carbon footprints. By implementing economic incentives that support plant-based businesses, governments can not only foster innovation and growth within the industry but also contribute to a more sustainable and environmentally friendly food system.

GLOBAL TRADE AND PLANT-BASED COMMODITIES

Global trade has played a significant role in the distribution and consumption of plant-based commodities around the world. As the demand for plant-based products has surged, international trade has facilitated the exchange of these goods across countries and continents. This has led to the growth of a global market for plant-based commodities, where producers can reach a wider consumer base and consumers can access a diverse range of products. The globalization of trade has allowed countries to specialize in the production of specific plant-based commodities, taking advantage of their comparative advantages in terms of climate, resources, and expertise. South American countries such as Brazil and Argentina have become major exporters of soybeans and soy products, while Southeast Asian countries dominate the market for palm oil. The expansion of global trade in plant-based commodities has also raised concerns about the environmental and social impacts of production, particularly in regions where natural ecosystems are being depleted to make way for large-scale agriculture. As the demand for plant-based products continues to rise, it is crucial to ensure that global trade remains sustainable and equitable, promoting both the well-being of people and the planet.

THE ROLE OF PLANT-BASED DIETS IN SUSTAINABILITY

The role of plant-based diets in sustainability has gained significant attention. Advocates argue that transitioning towards plant-based diets not only has numerous health benefits but also plays a crucial role in preserving the environment. Plant-based diets require significantly less land, water, and other resources compared to animal-based diets. Livestock farming is a resource-intensive industry that leads to deforestation, water pollution, and greenhouse gas emissions. By embracing plant-based diets, individuals can reduce their carbon footprint and contribute to the fight against climate change. Plant-based diets promote biodiversity and prevent the loss of wildlife habitats. The overconsumption of animal products has been linked to various environmental challenges, including land degradation and species extinction. Plant-based diets, on the other hand, support sustainable agriculture practices that prioritize soil health and conservation. By choosing plant-based options, individuals can actively participate in the shift towards a more sustainable and environmentally-friendly food system. Through conscious dietary decisions, individuals can make a significant impact on the long-term health and well-being of the planet.

CONTRIBUTION TO SUSTAINABLE DEVELOPMENT GOALS

The plant-based revolution has the potential to make a significant contribution to sustainable development goals. The adoption of a plant-based diet can directly address several of these goals, including the promotion of health and well-being, the reduction of greenhouse gas emissions, and the conservation of biodiversity. Plant-based diets have been linked to a lower risk of chronic diseases such as heart disease, diabetes, and certain types of cancer. By reducing the consumption of animal products, individuals can also reduce their carbon footprint and contribute to the mitigation of climate change. Livestock production is one of the leading causes of greenhouse gas emissions, deforestation, and water pollution. The expansion of industrial animal agriculture often leads to the destruction of natural habitats and the loss of biodiversity. By shifting towards a plant-based diet, individuals can help protect and restore ecosystems, preserve natural resources, and ensure the sustainability of our planet for future generations. Thus, the plant-based revolution has the potential to be a powerful tool in achieving the sustainable development goals.

PLANT-BASED DIETS AND THE CIRCULAR ECONOMY

Plant-based diets play a crucial role in the circular economy. The circular economy is an economic system aimed at minimizing waste and maximizing resource efficiency. In this system, materials are reused, recycled, or repurposed to create a closed-loop cycle. Plant-based diets align seamlessly with the principles of the circular economy as they promote the use of renewable resources and reduce waste. Unlike traditional meat-based diets, which heavily rely on animal agriculture and contribute to deforestation, climate change, and water pollution, plant-based diets rely on plants, which are highly renewable and require fewer resources to produce. By choosing plant-based diets, individuals actively contribute to reducing their ecological footprint and minimizing waste generation. The by-products of plant-based foods, such as vegetable scraps, can be composted and used as environmental-friendly fertilizers. The integration of plant-based diets into the circular economy can lead to a more sustainable and resource-efficient food system, benefiting both human health and the environment.

LONG-TERM ENVIRONMENTAL BENEFITS

One of the most compelling reasons to embrace a plant-based diet is the long-term environmental benefits it offers. Animal agriculture is a significant contributor to greenhouse gas emissions, deforestation, and water pollution. By shifting towards a plant-based diet, individuals can reduce their carbon footprint and help mitigate climate change. Plant-based diets require fewer resources and emit fewer greenhouse gases compared to animal-based diets. Embracing plant-based alternatives to animal products can help conserve natural resources such as land and water. Livestock farming requires vast amounts of land for grazing and growing animal feed, leading to deforestation and habitat destruction. Animal agriculture is a major consumer of freshwater, contributing to water scarcity and pollution. By choosing plant-based options, individuals can play a crucial role in preserving biodiversity and protecting our ecosystems. It is important to note that the long-term environmental benefits of a plant-based diet extend beyond reducing greenhouse gas emissions and conserving resources. They also encompass promoting sustainable farming practices, reducing waste, and fostering a more resilient and sustainable food system.

THE SOCIAL DYNAMICS OF FOOD CHOICES

The social dynamics of food choices are intricately woven into the fabric of our society. There has been a growing movement towards plant-based diets as individuals become more conscious of the environmental and health impacts of their food choices. The emergence of this plant-based revolution is reshaping the way we view food and transforming the dining landscape. One of the key factors driving this change is the increased accessibility and diversity of plant-based options, which cater to a wide range of preferences and dietary restrictions. Social media and online communities have played a significant role in popularizing plant-based diets, providing a platform for individuals to share recipes, stories, and advice, fostering a sense of community and support. It is important to acknowledge that the adoption of plant-based diets is not solely motivated by personal health or environmental concerns. For many, food choices are laden with cultural, ethical, and socioeconomic implications. The social dynamics of food choices must be comprehensively examined, taking into account a myriad of factors that shape our dietary preferences and practices.

PEER INFLUENCE AND DIETARY DECISIONS

Peer influence plays a significant role in shaping dietary decisions, especially among college students. The college years are a critical period where individuals are exposed to new experiences and influences, including those of their peers. It is not uncommon for students to adopt the eating habits of their friends and acquaintances, whether consciously or subconsciously. This phenomenon has been observed particularly in the context of vegetarian and vegan diets, which have gained considerable popularity in recent years. Social connections and group norms can strongly influence individuals' dietary choices, as students tend to seek acceptance and identify with their peer group. The availability and accessibility of plant-based options on campuses also contribute to the influence of peers on dietary decisions. As students witness their peers making dietary changes and experiencing the associated benefits, such as improved health and environmental consciousness, they may be motivated to adopt similar eating patterns. Peer influence, therefore, has a powerful impact on dietary decisions among college students, making it crucial for educational institutions to recognize and support healthy food choices in order to promote overall well-being.

THE ROLE OF FAMILY IN ADOPTING PLANT-BASED DIETS

Family serves as a social support system and plays a significant role in shaping individual dietary choices. Research suggests that family members have a direct influence on one another's eating habits, and it is through these familial interactions that the adoption of a plant-based diet can be facilitated. First and foremost, the family environment can promote the sharing of information and knowledge about plant-based foods. This exchange can serve as a catalyst for family members to try new recipes, experiment with different cooking methods, and explore alternative food sources. Family meals provide an opportunity for socialization and bonding, cultivating a sense of togetherness that can reinforce the adoption and maintenance of a plant-based diet. Family members can act as role models and encourage one another to make healthier food choices, which can help in overcoming barriers and challenges associated with transitioning to a plant-based lifestyle. The involvement and support of the family are crucial in successfully adopting and sustaining a plant-based diet.

SOCIAL IDENTITY AND FOOD CONSUMPTION

Social identity plays a crucial role in determining food consumption patterns. There has been a significant shift towards plant-based diets, driven by various social factors. One such factor is the growing awareness of the environmental impact of meat and dairy industries. Individuals who identify as environmentalists or are part of certain social movements, such as veganism or vegetarianism, tend to adopt plant-based diets as a means of reducing their carbon footprint. Social identity also influences food choices through cultural norms and beliefs. Individuals who identify with certain cultural or religious groups may be more inclined to follow dietary restrictions or preferences associated with their identity. The rise of social media platforms has allowed individuals to form online communities with shared ideals and values, including food choices. These communities reinforce and validate specific dietary practices, thereby influencing an individual's food consumption patterns. Social identity is a significant determinant of food consumption, as it shapes individuals' environmental consciousness, cultural influences, and affinity towards specific social groups.

THE IMPACT ON SMALL FARMERS AND RURAL COMMUNITIES

The shift towards plant-based diets undoubtedly has a significant impact on small farmers and rural communities. Traditional agriculture, with its focus on livestock and animal products, has long been the backbone of these communities. The rise of plant-based alternatives has led to a decline in demand for animal products, resulting in financial strain on farmers who solely rely on livestock for their livelihood. The increasing popularity of plant-based diets has resulted in a decrease in the number of small-scale, family-owned farms as larger corporations dominate the market. This not only affects farmers themselves but also has wider implications for the rural communities that rely on agriculture as an economic driver. The shift towards plant-based diets has the potential to reshape rural landscapes. As small-scale livestock farms go out of business, the land they once occupied may be repurposed for alternative uses such as plant-based agriculture or renewable energy production. While this may pave the way for a more sustainable future, it also raises concerns about the impact on local economies and cultural heritage tied to traditional farming practices. Thus, it is crucial for policymakers and stakeholders to address and support the transition of small farmers and rural communities to ensure their resilience and empowerment amidst the plant-based revolution.

TRANSITIONING TO PLANT-BASED CROP PRODUCTION

With the ever-increasing global population and the escalating concerns over climate change, traditional methods of crop production are becoming increasingly unsustainable. Transitioning to plant-based crop production involves a shift towards cultivating crops that are primarily used for human consumption, as opposed to crops grown for animal feed or biofuels. This transition not only reduces our dependence on animal agriculture, which is a major contributor to greenhouse gas emissions and deforestation, but it also promotes the efficient use of resources such as water and land. Plant-based agriculture offers a multitude of health benefits, as it encourages the consumption of nutrient-rich fruits, vegetables, and whole grains. Plant-based crop production can play a crucial role in addressing food security issues, as it allows for greater food availability and diversity. Transitioning to plant-based crop production requires a comprehensive approach that includes policy changes, increased support for farmers, and the implementation of sustainable farming practices. Through collective efforts and innovative solutions, we can successfully transition to a more sustainable and plant-based agricultural system that benefits both the environment and human health.

ECONOMIC CHALLENGES AND OPPORTUNITIES

Another economic challenge that arises from the plant-based revolution is the potential impact on existing industries, particularly the meat and dairy industries. As consumers are increasingly turning to plant-based alternatives, traditional meat and dairy companies may face declining demand for their products. This can lead to job loss and economic instability in regions heavily reliant on these industries. This challenge also presents opportunities for adaptation and growth. Companies in the meat and dairy industry can choose to capitalize on the growing demand for plant-based alternatives by diversifying their product lines or investing in research and development to improve the taste and texture of plant-based products. New businesses have emerged in response to the plant-based revolution, such as plant-based meat manufacturers and vegan food startups, creating job opportunities and invigorating the economy. The plant-based revolution also has the potential to create a more sustainable and efficient food system, leading to cost savings in areas such as healthcare and environmental conservation. As these economic challenges and opportunities continue to unfold, it is crucial for policymakers and industries to adapt and navigate these changes in order to ensure a smooth transition and maximize the benefits of the plant-based revolution.

COMMUNITY-LED INITIATIVES AND SUPPORT SYSTEMS

With the rising demand for plant-based options, communities have come together to create organizations, campaigns, and resources that educate and support individuals in their transition to a plant-based lifestyle. These initiatives provide a sense of belonging and community, making the journey more accessible and enjoyable. Websites and social media platforms offer recipes, meal plans, and tips to help individuals navigate the challenges of veganism. Community-led campaigns raise awareness about the environmental and ethical implications of animal agriculture, fostering a sense of social responsibility. These initiatives also connect individuals with local farmers, restaurants, and grocery stores that offer plant-based options, thereby expanding the accessibility and availability of plant-based foods. Community-led support systems, such as local vegan meetups, potlucks, and support groups, provide a space for individuals to share their experiences, ask questions, and find support from like-minded individuals. It is through these community-led initiatives and support systems that the plant-based revolution can gain momentum and become a sustainable way of life.

THE ROLE OF PLANT-BASED DIETS IN DISASTER RELIEF

The role of plant-based diets in disaster relief is a topic that is gaining increasing attention in today's world. As the frequency and intensity of natural disasters continue to rise, it is becoming clear that traditional relief efforts are not sufficient in addressing the long-term challenges posed by these calamities. Plant-based diets offer a sustainable and environmentally friendly solution to combat food insecurity during such crises. Apart from their low ecological footprint, plant-based diets are also rich in essential nutrients, providing a well-balanced and healthy source of sustenance for affected individuals. The cultivation of plant-based foods requires less water and land as compared to animal-based agriculture, making it an ideal choice in disaster-prone areas where resources are already limited. This approach also fosters community resilience and self-sufficiency, as the emphasis on local and sustainable food production empowers individuals to take control of their own food security. By incorporating plant-based diets into disaster relief efforts, humanitarian organizations can not only address immediate hunger but also contribute to long-term food sustainability and resilience in affected communities.

EFFICIENCY OF PLANT-BASED FOOD DISTRIBUTION IN CRISES

A key advantage of plant-based food distribution in times of crises is its efficiency. Plant-based food distribution systems have been shown to be more streamlined and cost-effective compared to traditional methods. The production and distribution of plant-based food products require fewer resources, such as water and land, making it an environmentally sustainable option. The transportation and storage of plant-based food items are often less complex, as they have longer shelf lives and do not require extensive refrigeration. In times of crises when supply chains may be disrupted, the efficiency of plant-based food distribution becomes even more relevant. With the ability to grow crops quickly and in large quantities, plant-based food production can be ramped up in response to increased demand. The flexibility of plant-based food production allows for a wider variety of products to be distributed, ensuring a diverse and nutritious diet for individuals affected by crises. The efficiency of plant-based food distribution makes it a viable solution in times of crises, offering sustainable and accessible nutrition to those in need.

NUTRITIONAL ADEQUACY IN EMERGENCY SITUATIONS

In emergency situations, ensuring nutritional adequacy becomes crucial as access to food might be limited or disrupted. Plant-based diets have the potential to address this challenge as they can provide the necessary nutrients while reducing reliance on animal agriculture, which is resource-intensive and environmentally unsustainable. A well-planned plant-based diet includes a variety of whole grains, legumes, fruits, vegetables, nuts, and seeds, which are rich sources of fiber, vitamins, minerals, and antioxidants. These nutrient-dense foods can help protect against malnutrition and deficiency-related diseases. Plant-based diets contribute to food security by promoting sustainable farming practices, reducing deforestation, and preserving water resources. The cultivation of plant-based foods requires less land and resources compared to animal agriculture, making them more feasible in emergency situations where there may be limited resources. It is crucial to ensure that plant-based diets in emergency situations are nutritionally adequate and provide appropriate protein, iron, calcium, zinc, vitamin B12, and omega-3 fatty acids, which are commonly found in animal products. Adequately addressing nutritional needs in emergency situations requires careful planning, cooperation between governments, aid agencies, and nutrition experts to ensure the availability, accessibility, and affordability of diverse plant-based food sources.

PLANT-BASED DIETS AS A SOLUTION TO FOOD AID DEPENDENCY

One potential solution to addressing food aid dependency is the adoption of plant-based diets. There has been a growing body of research supporting the health and environmental benefits of plant-based diets. By promoting the consumption of fruits, vegetables, whole grains, and legumes, plant-based diets can provide essential nutrients while minimizing the reliance on food aid. Plant-based diets have been associated with lower risks of chronic diseases, such as heart disease, diabetes, and certain types of cancer. This is particularly relevant in regions with limited access to healthcare, where the prevention of such diseases is crucial. Plant-based diets have a lower environmental impact, as they require less land, water, and energy compared to animal-based diets. By reducing the demand for animal agriculture, plant-based diets can contribute to mitigating the negative effects of livestock farming on climate change and deforestation. The promotion of plant-based diets as a sustainable and nutritious alternative could potentially alleviate the burden of food aid dependency and lead to improved health outcomes and environmental sustainability.

THE INTERSECTION WITH ANIMAL RIGHTS MOVEMENTS

The plant-based revolution has not only transformed the way we perceive and consume food but has also brought about a significant intersection with animal rights movements. As more individuals adopt a plant-based lifestyle, they become increasingly aware of the ethical implications of animal agriculture. Animal rights movements advocate for the fair and just treatment of animals, arguing that animals have inherent rights that should be protected. By adopting a plant-based diet, individuals align themselves with the principles of animal rights, as they actively choose to abstain from consuming products derived from animal exploitation. The plant-based revolution has empowered animal rights activists to push for legislative changes and advancements in animal welfare. These movements work towards promoting the recognition and protection of animal rights, challenging the industry's current practices and seeking alternatives that are more compassionate and sustainable. The plant-based revolution has therefore provided a platform for animal rights advocates to amplify their message and gain greater support for their cause, ultimately leading to a more compassionate and conscious society.

COLLABORATION BETWEEN PLANT-BASED AND ANIMAL RIGHTS ADVOCATES

Plant-based and animal rights advocates saw little common ground for collaboration in the past due to differences in their priorities and approaches. In recent years, there has been a growing recognition that collaboration between these two groups is essential for promoting a more sustainable and ethical food system. Both plant-based and animal rights advocates share a common goal of reducing animal suffering and promoting a more compassionate society. Plant-based advocates, with their focus on promoting the consumption of plant-based foods, can provide valuable support to animal rights advocates by creating a demand for cruelty-free products and encouraging individuals to adopt a plant-based diet. On the other hand, animal rights advocates, with their strong ethical stance against animal exploitation, can help plant-based advocates in raising awareness about the negative environmental and ethical impacts of animal agriculture. By working together, these two groups can create a powerful movement that not only addresses the ethical concerns surrounding animal rights but also the ecological concerns associated with animal agriculture. This collaboration has the potential to bring about transformative change in our food system, leading to a more sustainable and compassionate future.

SHARED GOALS AND STRATEGIES

Given the interconnectedness of various global issues, collaboration among diverse stakeholders is imperative to address the complex challenges associated with transitioning to a plant-based diet. Building coalitions and partnerships can provide a platform for diverse actors, such as governments, non-governmental organizations, and industry leaders, to collectively work towards common goals. These goals may include promoting public health, reducing greenhouse gas emissions, or preserving biodiversity. By aligning their strategies and pooling their resources, these stakeholders can maximize their impact and empower individuals to make sustainable choices. Shared goals create a sense of urgency and legitimacy, which can help garner support from policymakers and the wider society. Through collective action, it is possible to drive systemic change and create a lasting shift towards a plant-based food system. The success of the plant-based revolution rests on the ability of different actors to cooperate and share a common vision for a more sustainable future.

THE IMPACT ON LEGISLATION AND ANIMAL WELFARE STANDARDS

The impact of the plant-based revolution extends beyond just shifting consumer preferences and economic markets. It has also had a significant influence on legislation and animal welfare standards. As the demand for plant-based products continues to rise, lawmakers and regulatory bodies have recognized the need to update and strengthen existing laws and regulations to better protect animal welfare. This includes measures to improve living conditions for animals on farms and in slaughterhouses, as well as stricter regulations on labeling and transparency in the food industry. The plant-based revolution has encouraged the introduction of new legislation to promote and support the growth of alternative protein sources. This includes financial incentives for companies and individuals involved in sustainable farming practices, as well as policies that encourage the inclusion of plant-based options in schools, hospitals, and other public institutions. The plant-based revolution has brought about important changes in legislation and animal welfare standards, driving not only consumer behavior but also the legal and regulatory landscape surrounding animal rights and welfare.

THE ROLE OF PLANT-BASED DIETS IN CULTURAL PRESERVATION

In the modern world, where globalization and industrialization have contributed to the homogenization of cultures, there is a growing need to preserve and protect the diversity of cultural practices. One way to achieve this is through the promotion of plant-based diets. Plant-based diets have been an integral part of many cultures around the world for centuries. They not only provide sustenance but also carry deep cultural significance. By embracing these diets, communities can preserve their unique culinary traditions, rituals, and knowledge about the local environment. In Indian culture, vegetarianism is deeply rooted in religious and spiritual beliefs. It is also associated with the concept of ahimsa, or non-violence, and the belief that all living beings deserve respect and compassion. Similarly, in Mexican cuisine, corn, beans, and chili peppers hold enormous cultural value and are essential components of traditional dishes like tortillas and mole sauces. By promoting plant-based diets, societies can safeguard their cultural heritage, maintain their connection to the natural world, and foster respect for the environment and all living beings.

ADAPTING TRADITIONAL DISHES TO PLANT-BASED ALTERNATIVES

The concept of adapting traditional dishes to plant-based alternatives has gained significant traction in recent years, as more individuals embrace a plant-based lifestyle. With a growing awareness of the detrimental effects of animal agriculture on the environment and personal health, many have made the conscious decision to replace animal products with plant-based alternatives. One of the key ways to achieve this transition is through the adaptation of traditional dishes. By substituting animal-based ingredients with plant-based counterparts, individuals can continue to enjoy the flavors and textures they are familiar with, while supporting their ethical and environmental values. Classic dishes like lasagna can be made using plant-based minced meat substitutes and vegan cheese, resulting in a satisfying and guilt-free meal. Similarly, traditional favorites like burgers can be crafted from plant-based patties, offering the same mouthwatering experience without the reliance on animal products. Adapting traditional dishes to plant-based alternatives not only allows individuals to remain connected to their cultural culinary heritage but also encourages innovation and creativity in the realm of plant-based cooking.

CULTURAL HERITAGE AND PLANT-BASED CUISINE

Cultural heritage plays a significant role in the development and evolution of plant-based cuisine. Throughout history, various cultures have cultivated a profound connection with their natural surroundings, allowing them to incorporate local plants and produce into their traditional dishes. This cultural heritage not only reflects the land's biodiversity but also aligns with sustainable practices. In Asian cuisine, ingredients like tofu, tempeh, and soy sauce have been used for centuries as a viable source of protein. In Indian cuisine, lentils and legumes are staple ingredients that provide essential nutrients and are integral to vegetarian and vegan meals. Cultural festivals and rituals often revolve around plant-based dishes, showcasing the importance of sustainable options in these events. The fusion of cultural heritage and plant-based cuisine not only serves to preserve traditional recipes but also as a means of promoting a healthier lifestyle and an environmentally conscious approach to eating. By understanding and celebrating cultural heritage, individuals can embrace the rich diversity of plant-based cuisine and reap the benefits it offers.

THE BALANCE BETWEEN INNOVATION AND TRADITION

On one hand, innovation drives the development and advancement of plant-based products that can mimic the taste, texture, and nutritional composition of animal-based foods. This creative approach allows for the expansion of the market to appeal to a broader consumer base, including those who are initially skeptical of a plant-based diet. The introduction of innovative products such as plant-based burgers that closely resemble their traditional meat counterparts have gained popularity among both vegetarians and meat-eaters alike. On the other hand, tradition plays a significant role in maintaining cultural practices, culinary heritage, and a sense of identity associated with food. Striking a balance between innovation and tradition is essential to ensure the acceptance and sustainability of the plant-based revolution. This can be achieved by incorporating plant-based ingredients into traditional recipes, promoting the consumption of locally sourced plant-based foods, and encouraging a holistic approach to dietary choices that values sustainability and cultural diversity. Embracing both innovation and tradition enables a synergistic transformation towards a more plant-based future.

THE IMPACT ON GLOBAL FOOD SECURITY

With the increasing global population and the challenges posed by climate change, ensuring food security has become a pressing issue. XXXV. The impact on global food security can be significant through the adoption of plant-based diets. Plant-based diets have the potential to address both the issue of food scarcity and environmental sustainability. Currently, livestock production accounts for a significant amount of greenhouse gas emissions, deforestation, and water pollution. By shifting towards a plant-based diet, these negative impacts can be mitigated. Plant-based diets can utilize land more efficiently, as it takes significantly more resources to produce animal-based products compared to plant-based ones. This transition could potentially free up land, making it available for other agricultural purposes or reforestation efforts. Plant-based diets offer a more sustainable solution to feeding the growing global population compared to traditional meat-based diets. With the adoption of plant-based diets, countries can decrease their reliance on resource-intensive animal agriculture, consequently reducing the pressure on land, water, and energy resources, thereby significantly contributing to improving global food security.

THE ROLE OF PLANT-BASED DIETS IN FEEDING A GROWING POPULATION

As the global population continues to grow, the demand for food is also on the rise. Plant-based diets offer a potential solution to this challenge, as they can provide sustainable and nutritious food sources. Unlike traditional animal-based agriculture, plant-based agriculture requires less land, water, and energy inputs. By shifting towards a plant-based diet, we can reduce the strain on our planet's resources and mitigate the negative environmental impacts associated with animal agriculture, such as deforestation and greenhouse gas emissions. Plant-based diets can offer health benefits, as they are often rich in essential nutrients, fiber, and antioxidants. As such, promoting and adopting plant-based diets can help address both the sustainability and health concerns of a growing population. It is important to recognize that the transition to plant-based diets should be done in a culturally sensitive manner, taking into consideration the diverse dietary traditions and food preferences of different populations.

REDUCING DEPENDENCY ON ANIMAL PROTEIN FOR FOOD SECURITY

The current system of industrialized animal agriculture not only contributes significantly to greenhouse gas emissions and deforestation but also requires vast amounts of land, water, and energy. The consumption of animal protein has been linked to various chronic health problems such as heart disease, obesity, and some forms of cancer. Transitioning to a more plant-based diet offers an opportunity to increase food security by reducing the strain on natural resources and improving public health outcomes. Plant-based protein sources, such as legumes, nuts, and seeds, are not only more sustainable and less resource-intensive but also contain essential nutrients and are often cheaper to produce. By promoting plant-based options through increased availability, affordability, and education, societies can reduce their reliance on animal protein while ensuring food security for a growing global population. This shift can empower individuals to make healthier choices, ultimately leading to improved overall well-being.

THE POTENTIAL FOR PLANT-BASED DIETS TO MITIGATE HUNGER

As the global population continues to grow, there is an urgent need to find sustainable solutions to alleviate hunger and food insecurity. Plant-based diets offer a promising avenue to address this issue, as they require significantly fewer resources to produce compared to animal-based diets. According to research, plant-based diets have the potential to feed a much larger population with limited resources. This is because plant-based foods, such as grains, legumes, and vegetables, can be grown more efficiently and yield a higher caloric output per unit of land. The production of plant-based foods generates fewer greenhouse gas emissions and consumes less water, making them more environmentally sustainable. Transitioning towards plant-based diets can free up land that is currently used for animal agriculture, which can then be repurposed for growing crops to feed people directly. In light of these advantages, promoting plant-based diets not only has the potential to improve health and reduce environmental degradation but also to mitigate hunger on a global scale.

THE ROLE OF PERSONAL RESPONSIBILITY AND CHOICE

Personal responsibility and choice play a pivotal role in the pursuit of a plant-based lifestyle. The decision to adopt such a diet is a matter of individual choice, driven by personal values, ethical concerns, and health considerations. The adoption of a plant-based diet requires a conscious effort to take responsibility for one's own health and well-being. It is not a decision that can be forced or imposed upon an individual. Rather, it is a choice that must be made willingly and with the understanding of its potential impact on one's lifestyle and overall health. Personal responsibility entails not only making the initial choice to follow a plant-based diet but also the ongoing commitment to adhere to it. This commitment involves making informed decisions about food choices, sourcing organic and sustainable products, and actively seeking out plant-based alternatives. It also necessitates being accountable for one's own actions, recognizing that personal choices have far-reaching consequences for oneself, animals, and the environment. Personal responsibility and choice are integral components of the plant-based revolution, empowering individuals to make conscious decisions that positively impact their own health and the world around them.

INDIVIDUAL IMPACT THROUGH DIETARY CHOICES

By adopting a plant-based diet, individuals can make a significant positive impact on their health, the environment, and animal welfare. Firstly, people who consume a plant-based diet tend to have lower rates of obesity, heart disease, diabetes, and certain types of cancer. Consuming a diet high in fruits, vegetables, whole grains, and legumes provides essential nutrients and antioxidants that promote overall health and wellbeing. Adopting a plant-based diet helps reduce carbon emissions, water usage, and deforestation, which are major contributors to climate change. The livestock industry is responsible for a significant percentage of greenhouse gas emissions, and by reducing or eliminating animal products from one's diet, individuals can decrease their carbon footprint. Transitioning to a plant-based diet helps combat animal cruelty by refusing to support industries that prioritize profit over animal welfare. By making conscious dietary choices, individuals can make a powerful and positive impact on their own health, the planet, and the wellbeing of animals.

THE ETHICS OF PERSONAL CONSUMPTION

As individuals increasingly embrace a plant-based lifestyle, it becomes necessary to examine the moral implications of our personal consumption choices. One of the key ethical concerns relates to the environmental impact of animal agriculture. The production of animal-based food not only contributes to deforestation and water pollution but also generates substantial greenhouse gas emissions. By transitioning to a plant-based diet, individuals can significantly reduce their ecological footprint. The ethical dimension extends beyond the environmental realm. Factory farming, for instance, raises concerns about animal welfare and the potential mistreatment of animals. Choosing to consume plant-based products allows individuals to align their values with their actions and reject systems that prioritize profit over the well-being of living beings. Nonetheless, the ethics of personal consumption require a nuanced approach as other factors such as food accessibility, cultural practices, and individual health considerations must also be taken into account. Examining the ethics of personal consumption within the context of the plant-based revolution illuminates the importance of considering the environmental and ethical consequences of our choices and taking responsibility for our impact on the world.

EMPOWERMENT THROUGH INFORMED FOOD DECISIONS

As society becomes increasingly aware of the detrimental effects of animal agriculture on the environment and personal health, individuals are taking charge of their own well-being by making conscious choices about the food they consume. Informed food decisions are those that are based on reliable information and a deep understanding of the implications of our dietary choices. By educating themselves about the benefits of a plant-based diet, individuals become empowered to make choices that align with their values, health goals, and environmental concerns. This empowerment extends to advocating for change on a larger scale, such as supporting local farmers markets, demanding sustainable and ethical food options in schools and workplaces, and encouraging restaurants to offer more plant-based menu choices. Informed food decisions not only improve individual health but also contribute to building a sustainable and compassionate food system for future generations. Thus, by taking charge of what we put on our plates, we have the power to shape a healthier, more sustainable world.

THE INTERSECTION OF PLANT-BASED DIETS AND FAIR TRADE

As the popularity of plant-based diets continues to grow, so does the demand for products that align with ethical and sustainable practices. One such practice is fair trade, which aims to provide better trading conditions and promote sustainability for producers in developing countries. The intersection of plant-based diets and fair trade presents a unique opportunity to create a more just and sustainable food system. Plant-based diets inherently prioritize the consumption of fruits, vegetables, grains, and other plant-based products, making them compatible with fair trade principles. By choosing plant-based alternatives sourced from fair trade producers, individuals can contribute to the well-being of farmers and workers, while also reducing the environmental impact of their food choices. Fair trade ensures that farming practices are environmentally friendly, promoting biodiversity and reducing the use of harmful chemicals. By embracing a plant-based diet and supporting fair trade, we can work towards a more equitable and sustainable future, one where both human welfare and the health of the planet are prioritized.

ENSURING ETHICAL SOURCING OF PLANT-BASED INGREDIENTS

As more consumers turn to plant-based diets for health or ethical reasons, companies must take responsibility for the impact of their ingredient sourcing on both humans and the environment. Ethical sourcing encompasses various aspects, including fair labor practices, sustainable farming methods, and protection of biodiversity. Firstly, companies should ensure that their suppliers adhere to fair labor practices, treating workers with dignity and fair compensation. This includes providing safe working conditions and fair wages, as well as safeguarding against child labor and exploitation. Secondly, sustainable farming methods should be employed to minimize negative environmental impacts. This may involve organic farming practices, such as avoiding synthetic pesticides and fertilizers, and protecting soil health. Protecting biodiversity through responsible sourcing is crucial. Utilizing diverse plant species instead of monocultures can help preserve ecosystems and prevent the loss of endangered species. By prioritizing ethical sourcing, companies can contribute to a more sustainable and equitable plant-based revolution.

THE RELATIONSHIP BETWEEN FAIR TRADE AND FOOD QUALITY

Fair trade and food quality have a close relationship that is gaining increasing attention in the context of the plant-based revolution. As consumers become more concerned about the ethical and environmental implications of their food choices, they are looking for products that not only ensure fair compensation for farmers but also deliver high-quality, nutritious food. Fair trade certification guarantees that farmers receive fair prices for their products, and this often translates into better quality food. Fair trade focuses on sustainable and responsible production practices, which can result in higher nutritional content and better taste in food products. Fair trade encourages the use of organic and environmentally friendly farming methods, which further enhances the quality of the food. By choosing fair trade products, consumers can not only support fair compensation for farmers but also enjoy food that is both ethically produced and of superior quality. The relationship between fair trade and food quality demonstrates the potential for creating a more sustainable and equitable food system while still meeting the demand for high-quality products.

THE IMPACT ON PRODUCERS IN DEVELOPING COUNTRIES

One of the key impacts of the plant-based revolution is felt by producers in developing countries. As consumer demands for plant-based products soar, there is an increased demand for ingredients such as soybeans, rice, and various types of vegetables that are predominantly cultivated in these developing nations. This surge in demand presents a significant economic opportunity for farmers and agricultural businesses in these countries, as it allows them to expand their production and meet the international demand. Not only does this lead to increased employment opportunities for locals, but it also contributes to the overall economic growth of these nations. As the global market for plant-based products expands, it encourages producers in developing countries to adopt more sustainable farming practices to meet the increased demand. This shift towards sustainable agriculture has a positive impact on the environment, as it promotes the maintenance of soil quality, reduces water usage, and minimizes chemical inputs. The plant-based revolution not only benefits producers in developing countries economically but also encourages them to adopt more sustainable farming practices for a greener future.

THE ROLE OF PLANT-BASED DIETS IN PREVENTATIVE MEDICINE

There has been a growing interest in plant-based diets and their potential role in preventative medicine. Research has shown that adopting a plant-based diet can have numerous health benefits, reducing the risk of chronic diseases such as heart disease, type 2 diabetes, and certain types of cancer. Plant-based diets are typically low in saturated fats and high in dietary fiber, antioxidants, and phytochemicals, which contribute to their protective effects. Studies have also demonstrated that plant-based diets can help maintain a healthy weight, decrease inflammation, and improve overall gut health. Plant-based diets have been associated with a reduced risk of developing metabolic syndrome, a cluster of conditions that increase the risk of heart disease, stroke, and diabetes. These compelling findings have led to a growing recognition of the importance of plant-based diets in preventative medicine, with many health organizations advocating for the inclusion of more plant-based foods in daily dietary patterns. While further research is needed to fully understand the mechanisms underlying these effects, the current evidence strongly supports the role of plant-based diets in promoting long-term health and preventing chronic diseases.

THE USE OF PLANT-BASED DIETS IN DISEASE PREVENTION

One of the most notable benefits of plant-based diets is their potential to prevent the onset of various diseases. Research has consistently shown that individuals who consume a predominantly plant-based diet have a lower risk of developing chronic conditions such as cardiovascular disease, type 2 diabetes, and certain types of cancer. This is primarily due to the high levels of fiber, antioxidants, and phytochemicals present in plant foods. Fiber, for instance, is known to lower cholesterol levels, regulate blood sugar levels, and promote healthy digestion. Antioxidants help combat oxidative stress and inflammation, key factors in the development of chronic diseases. Phytochemicals, on the other hand, have been found to possess anti-cancer properties and can help inhibit the growth of cancer cells. The avoidance of animal products in plant-based diets reduces the intake of unhealthy saturated and trans fats, which are associated with an increased risk of heart disease. Embracing a plant-based diet can therefore serve as a powerful tool in disease prevention, offering individuals the opportunity to improve their overall health and well-being.

INTEGRATING NUTRITION EDUCATION INTO MEDICAL TRAINING

Historically, medical education has focused primarily on pharmacology and interventions, leaving a significant gap in the knowledge of healthcare professionals regarding the impact of nutrition on disease prevention and management. Recent research has highlighted the integral role of nutrition in the pathogenesis of chronic diseases such as obesity, hypertension, and diabetes. Consequently, there is a growing emphasis on preventive medicine and lifestyle modifications, including dietary changes, to improve health outcomes. By integrating nutrition education into medical training, future healthcare professionals can develop a comprehensive understanding of how diet impacts health, allowing them to provide evidence-based dietary guidance to their patients. This paradigm shift in medical education will not only address the lack of nutrition knowledge but also empower healthcare professionals to effectively promote and support plant-based diets, which have been scientifically proven to reduce the risk of chronic diseases and improve overall health and well-being.

CASE STUDIES OF PLANT-BASED DIETS IN MEDICAL TREATMENT

One compelling aspect of the plant-based revolution is the growing number of case studies indicating the potential of plant-based diets in medical treatment. These studies demonstrate that adopting a plant-based diet can have significant positive effects on various health conditions. A case study published in the Journal of the American Heart Association showed that a plant-based diet can effectively reduce the risk of cardiovascular diseases. Another study conducted by the Physicians Committee for Responsible Medicine found that plant-based diets can be beneficial in managing type 2 diabetes. A case study published in the Journal of the Academy of Nutrition and Dietetics showed that plant-based diets can help improve bone health and reduce the risk of osteoporosis. These case studies provide empirical evidence that supports the argument for incorporating plant-based diets into medical treatment plans. They highlight the potential of plant-based diets to not only prevent but also reverse various chronic illnesses, making them a valuable addition to the field of medicine.

THE IMPACT ON THE FISHING INDUSTRY

The rise of the plant-based revolution has had a profound impact on the fishing industry. As more and more consumers are turning towards plant-based alternatives for their dietary needs, the demand for fish and seafood has significantly decreased. This shift in consumer preferences has led to a decline in fishing activities and a decrease in fish stocks worldwide. Fishing communities that heavily rely on the industry are experiencing economic hardships as a result. The decline in fish populations disrupts the delicate balance of marine ecosystems, affecting other organisms that depend on these fish for survival. The fishing industry itself is facing increasing scrutiny for its environmental practices, such as overfishing and destructive fishing methods. The plant-based revolution has thus prompted calls for more sustainable fishing practices and the preservation of marine ecosystems. To adapt and remain viable, some fishing communities are exploring alternative revenue streams, such as tourism or aquaculture. The long-term impact of the plant-based revolution on the fishing industry remains uncertain and poses significant challenges that need to be addressed for the sake of both fishing communities and the marine environment.

THE DECLINE IN DEMAND FOR SEAFOOD

One of the key contributors to this decline is the growing awareness about the environmental impacts of overfishing and unsustainable fishing practices. As consumers become more educated about the detrimental effects of these practices on marine ecosystems, they are increasingly opting for alternative sources of protein. Concerns about the presence of contaminants such as mercury and microplastics in seafood have also played a role in the decline in demand. The rise of plant-based diets has further accelerated this trend, as more individuals choose to adopt vegetarian or vegan lifestyles for health, ethical, and environmental reasons. The availability of a wide variety of plant-based alternatives, including mock seafood products, has made it easier for people to transition away from traditional seafood-based dishes. The COVID-19 pandemic and its disruptions to global supply chains have also had an impact on the decline in demand for seafood. As consumer preferences shift towards more sustainable and plant-based options, the seafood industry must adapt in order to remain viable in the face of changing dietary choices.

SUSTAINABLE ALTERNATIVES TO FISHING

One such alternative is the cultivation of underwater plants. By harnessing the power of photosynthesis, these plants not only serve as a source of food but also improve water quality and restore the ecological balance of marine ecosystems. This method involves the cultivation of various species such as kelp, seaweed, and algae in offshore areas. The plants not only provide a sustainable source of nutrition but also act as natural filters, absorbing excess nutrients and thereby preventing harmful algal blooms. The cultivation of underwater plants helps in carbon sequestration, assisting in the mitigation of climate change. Another sustainable alternative is the use of aquaculture systems. By farming fish in controlled environments, the negative impacts associated with overfishing and bycatch can be significantly reduced. Aquaculture systems can be designed to minimize the use of antibiotics and chemicals, thus producing healthier and more sustainable fish. The adoption of these sustainable alternatives offers a promising solution to the declining fish stocks and the degradation of marine ecosystems.

THE GROWTH OF PLANT-BASED SEAFOOD OPTIONS

As concerns about sustainability and animal welfare continue to rise, consumers are seeking alternatives to traditional seafood products. Plant-based seafood options offer a promising solution by providing a more sustainable and ethical choice. Companies like Good Catch and Sophie's Kitchen have emerged as leaders in this field, offering a variety of plant-based seafood products that mimic the taste and texture of popular seafood items such as fish, shrimp, and crab. These companies use innovative techniques and ingredients, such as a blend of legumes and algae, to recreate the flavors and textures of seafood without the negative environmental and ethical impacts associated with traditional fishing practices. The plant-based seafood market has witnessed significant growth in recent years, fueled by increasing consumer demand. This growth has been further supported by a growing number of restaurants and retailers that are incorporating plant-based seafood options into their menus and product offerings. The growth of plant-based seafood options represents a promising trend towards a more sustainable and ethical food system.

THE ROLE OF PLANT-BASED DIETS IN URBAN PLANNING

Urban planning plays a crucial role in addressing various societal challenges, including sustainable development, climate change, and public health. One aspect of urban planning that has gained increasing attention is the role of plant-based diets. Plant-based diets, characterized by the consumption of fruits, vegetables, whole grains, and legumes while minimizing or avoiding animal products, have been proven to have numerous benefits for both individuals and the environment. In the context of urban planning, promoting plant-based diets can help to create healthier and more sustainable cities. By encouraging the establishment of farmers markets, community gardens, and urban farms, urban planners can provide residents with easy access to fresh and affordable plant-based foods. Incorporating green spaces and parks into urban designs can not only contribute to the aesthetic appeal of cities but also provide opportunities for urban farming and community gardening. By integrating plant-based diets into urban planning strategies, cities can reduce their ecological footprint, combat climate change, and improve public health. The role of plant-based diets in urban planning is essential for creating livable and sustainable cities.

INCORPORATING FOOD GARDENS AND GREEN SPACES

In addition to the environmental benefits of a plant-based diet, incorporating food gardens and green spaces into our communities also provides numerous advantages. Food gardens promote sustainable living by allowing us to grow our own produce in an organic and eco-friendly manner. Not only does this reduce our reliance on conventional farming methods, which are often resource-intensive and contribute to water pollution, but it also helps to address food insecurity and access to fresh, healthy foods. Green spaces, on the other hand, have been proven to enhance our physical and mental well-being. They provide a tranquil and peaceful environment, offering a much-needed respite from the fast-paced and stressful nature of modern life. Green spaces promote biodiversity and contribute to a healthy ecosystem by supporting the presence of various plant and animal species. By incorporating food gardens and green spaces into our communities, we can foster a stronger connection with nature, improve our overall health, and create more sustainable and resilient communities.

URBAN POLICIES PROMOTING PLANT-BASED LIVING

One key aspect of the plant-based revolution lies in the implementation of urban policies that promote plant-based living. These policies are essential in creating sustainable and environmentally friendly cities. Firstly, urban policies can encourage the development of community gardens and urban farming initiatives. By allocating land and resources for these initiatives, cities can foster a stronger connection between residents and their food sources while promoting the consumption of plant-based products.

Secondly, these policies can provide incentives for the establishment of plant-based restaurants and cafes. By offering tax breaks or financial support, cities can motivate entrepreneurs to open businesses that exclusively serve plant-based cuisine, thus providing more options for individuals looking to adopt a plant-based lifestyle. Urban policies can also prioritize the integration of plant-based menus in public institutions such as schools and hospitals. By mandating the inclusion of plant-based options, cities can ensure that individuals have access to healthy and sustainable food choices in various settings. Urban policies play a crucial role in fostering a plant-based revolution by creating a supportive and accommodating environment for individuals seeking to adopt plant-based living.

THE DEVELOPMENT OF FOOD HUBS AND LOCAL MARKETS

A food hub is a collaborative network that brings together farmers, producers, and consumers to improve the availability and accessibility of local, sustainable food. These hubs facilitate the production, distribution, and marketing of plant-based products, creating a meaningful connection between producers and consumers. Local markets also play a crucial role in promoting sustainable food systems. They provide a platform for local farmers to sell their plant-based products directly to consumers, eliminating the need for intermediaries and reducing carbon emissions associated with long-distance transportation. Local markets foster community engagement and provide valuable opportunities for consumers to connect with the people who grow their food. By supporting food hubs and local markets, individuals can actively contribute to the growth of the plant-based revolution and promote a more sustainable and equitable food system. This development aligns with the increasing consumer demand for transparent and ethically sourced plant-based products, fostering healthier and more environmentally friendly choices.

THE ROLE OF PLANT-BASED DIETS IN REDUCING FOOD WASTE

Plant-based diets present a potential solution to the pressing global issue of food waste. The inefficiency of animal agriculture significantly contributes to the wastage of vast amounts of resources. According to the Food and Agriculture Organization, animal-based products require more land, water, and energy to produce compared to plant-based alternatives. By shifting towards plant-based diets, individuals can greatly reduce their ecological footprint and minimize the wastage of these resources. Plant-based diets offer the advantage of versatility and adaptability to a wide range of food sources. Unlike animal-based diets that heavily rely on specific animals and their products, plant-based diets can utilize a variety of fruits, vegetables, legumes, and grains that are accessible and abundant. This diversity in food sources promotes a more balanced and sustainable diet, reducing the reliance on specific crops and thus the potential for crop failures and food shortages. Embracing plant-based diets can not only help alleviate food waste but also contribute to a more sustainable and resilient food system.

THE EFFICIENCY OF PLANT-BASED FOOD PRODUCTION

Unlike animal agriculture, which requires vast amounts of land, water, and feed, plant-based food production is far more efficient and sustainable. It takes approximately 16 pounds of grain to produce just one pound of beef, resulting in a tremendous waste of resources. In contrast, plant-based foods can be grown using significantly less land and water. Plant-based diets have a lower carbon footprint, as the production and transportation of meat and dairy products contribute significantly to greenhouse gas emissions. Plant-based diets require fewer resources for cultivation, such as fossil fuels and synthetic fertilizers, reducing pollution and environmental degradation. By eliminating the middleman of animal agriculture, plant-based food production has the potential to address global food insecurity and alleviate hunger on a large scale. The efficiency of plant-based food production offers a sustainable and viable solution to feed the growing population while minimizing environmental impact.

COMPOSTING AND RECYCLING IN PLANT-BASED COMMUNITIES

Composting and recycling play a crucial role in promoting sustainability and environmental conservation within plant-based communities. By composting organic waste materials such as fruit and vegetable scraps, plant-based communities can generate nutrient-rich soil amendments for their gardens, reducing the need for synthetic fertilizers. This not only reduces waste but also fosters a closed-loop system wherein waste is converted into a valuable resource. Recycling practices are essential in plant-based communities to minimize the consumption of virgin resources and decrease the production of greenhouse gas emissions associated with the extraction and manufacturing processes. By utilizing recycling systems and promoting the use of recycled materials, plant-based communities can contribute to the circular economy model. This not only reduces environmental impacts but also encourages sustainable practices and conscious consumption. By incorporating composting and recycling practices into the fabric of plant-based communities, individuals can actively participate in mitigating climate change and promoting a harmonious relationship between human activities and the natural world.

REDUCING FOOD WASTE THROUGH CONSUMER EDUCATION

Reducing food waste is crucial in our quest for a sustainable future, and one effective way to achieve this is through consumer education. By increasing public awareness about the consequences of food waste, individuals can make more informed choices that minimize spoilage. Consumer education can be achieved through various channels, including educational campaigns, workshops, and community outreach programs. These initiatives can help consumers better understand the value of food and develop practical strategies to reduce waste. Consumers can learn about proper storage techniques, portion control, and creative ways to utilize leftovers. Consumer education can also shed light on the environmental impact of food waste, such as the production of greenhouse gases and deforestation. Armed with this knowledge, individuals are more likely to adopt sustainable practices such as composting and advocating for policies that promote waste reduction. In essence, consumer education plays a pivotal role in reducing food waste by empowering individuals with knowledge and fostering a sense of responsibility towards the environment.

THE ROLE OF PLANT-BASED DIETS IN WATER CONSERVATION

The issue of water scarcity has taken center stage globally as the limited freshwater resources become increasingly stressed. As economies and populations continue to grow, so does the demand for water-intensive activities such as agriculture and livestock rearing. One potential solution lies in the adoption of plant-based diets, which significantly reduce water consumption compared to animal-based diets. Research shows that the production of plant-based foods requires significantly less water compared to the production of meat and dairy products. It takes approximately 1,100 gallons of water to produce a single pound of beef, while the same amount of water can produce around 40 pounds of corn. The water footprint of plant-based diets is not limited to crop production but also includes the indirect water required for livestock feed. By shifting to plant-based diets, individuals can substantially reduce their water footprint and contribute to global water conservation efforts. Promoting and adopting plant-based diets should be considered a vital aspect of any sustainable water management strategy.

WATER FOOTPRINT OF PLANT-BASED VERSUS ANIMAL-BASED FOODS

A key component of the plant-based revolution is the recognition of the significant differences between the water footprints of plant-based and animal-based foods. As the production of animal-based foods requires extensive resources, including land, feed, and water, the water footprint of these products tends to be considerably larger compared to their plant-based counterparts. It has been estimated that producing one kilogram of beef requires approximately 15,415 liters of water, while growing one kilogram of wheat only necessitates around 1,250 liters. This stark contrast in water usage highlights the potential environmental benefits of shifting towards a plant-based diet. By reducing our consumption of animal-based products and instead focusing on incorporating more plant-based options into our diets, we can help conserve water resources and mitigate the water scarcity challenges that many regions of the world face. Adopting a plant-based diet not only benefits the environment but also offers numerous health advantages, including reduced risk of chronic diseases. Understanding and considering the water footprint of our food choices is crucial for promoting a sustainable and transformative plant-based revolution.

THE IMPACT ON WATER SCARCITY AND MANAGEMENT

Water scarcity and management are crucial topics to address in the context of the plant-based revolution. As the demand for plant-based products continues to rise, the impact on water resources cannot be ignored. Agriculture accounts for a significant portion of water usage globally, and the cultivation of crops for plant-based products requires substantial amounts of water. The shift towards a plant-based diet could potentially exacerbate water scarcity in regions already facing water stress. Effective water management becomes increasingly important as the demand for plant-based products increases. Efficient irrigation systems, water conservation strategies, and sustainable farming practices must be implemented to minimize water waste and ensure the long-term availability of water resources. Collaboration between policymakers, industries, and communities is necessary to develop comprehensive water management strategies that address the unique challenges presented by the plant-based revolution. By acknowledging the impact on water scarcity and adopting responsible water management practices, the plant-based revolution can contribute to a more sustainable and equitable future for all.

INNOVATIONS IN WATER-EFFICIENT PLANT-BASED FARMING

A growing concern over water scarcity and sustainable agriculture has led to innovations in water-efficient plant-based farming. As the world's population continues to rise, traditional agricultural practices are no longer sufficient to meet the demand for food production. Water is a critical resource for agriculture, and its scarcity poses a significant challenge to farmers. In response to this challenge, innovative farming techniques have emerged, such as hydroponics and precision farming. Hydroponics involves growing plants in a nutrient-rich solution, without soil, in a controlled environment. This method requires significantly less water compared to traditional farming practices, as the nutrient solution is recirculated and reused. Precision farming, on the other hand, involves using technology, such as sensors and data analysis, to optimize water usage and crop productivity. By precisely delivering water to plants based on their needs, farmers can minimize water wastage. These innovations not only contribute to water conservation but also increase crop yields and reduce the environmental impact of agriculture. As water scarcity becomes a pressing issue globally, further research and adoption of water-efficient plant-based farming techniques will be essential to ensure sustainable food production for future generations.

THE ROLE OF PLANT-BASED DIETS IN SOIL HEALTH

There has been a growing interest in the role of plant-based diets in soil health. Plant-based diets, which focus on consuming predominantly fruits, vegetables, grains, legumes, and nuts, have been shown to have several benefits when it comes to soil health. Firstly, these diets tend to promote sustainable agriculture practices, such as organic farming, which minimize the use of synthetic pesticides and fertilizers that can harm soil health. Secondly, plant-based diets often incorporate a diverse range of plant species, which can enhance biodiversity within the soil. This biodiversity is crucial for the maintenance of healthy soil ecosystems, as it promotes nutrient cycling and helps to control pests and diseases. Plant-based diets contribute to increased organic matter content in the soil due to the incorporation of plant residues and compost. This organic matter improves soil structure, water retention, and nutrient availability, ultimately leading to healthier and more fertile soils. The adoption of plant-based diets can play a vital role in supporting soil health and achieving sustainable agriculture practices.

THE BENEFITS OF PLANT-BASED AGRICULTURE FOR SOIL

One major advantage is that plant-based agriculture helps prevent soil erosion. The extensive root system of many plants helps hold the soil in place, reducing the likelihood of it being carried away by wind or water. Plant-based agriculture promotes soil fertility. Unlike animal agriculture, which often requires the use of chemical fertilizers and other additives that can degrade soil quality over time, plant-based agriculture relies on natural processes to enhance soil health. Plants draw nutrients from the soil, and when they die and decompose, they return those nutrients back into the earth. This cycle improves soil fertility and promotes the growth of microorganisms that are vital for nutrient availability to plants. Plant-based agriculture supports the creation of healthy soil ecosystems. By cultivating a diverse range of plant species, farmers can enhance biodiversity below the ground, which promotes the presence of beneficial insects, worms, and microorganisms. These organisms contribute to nutrient cycling, soil structure, and water retention, leading to healthier and more resilient soil.

CROP ROTATION AND SUSTAINABLE FARMING PRACTICES

Crop rotation is the practice of systematically growing different crops in the same area over the course of several seasons. By rotating crops, farmers can break the cycle of pests and diseases that target specific crops, thus reducing the need for chemical pesticides. By growing a variety of crops with different nutrient requirements, farmers can improve soil fertility and reduce the risk of soil degradation. Sustainable farming practices, such as organic farming and agroforestry, further enhance the benefits of crop rotation by minimizing the use of synthetic fertilizers and promoting biodiversity. These practices prioritize soil conservation and water management, which are crucial for ensuring the sustainability of agricultural systems. By adopting crop rotation and sustainable farming practices, farmers can minimize environmental impacts, preserve natural resources, and promote the health and well-being of both humans and ecosystems in an increasingly challenging climate. As the demand for sustainable and nutritious food rises, it is imperative that farmers and policymakers prioritize and invest in these practices to ensure a more resilient and sustainable future for agriculture.

THE PREVENTION OF SOIL EROSION AND DEGRADATION

In addition to its numerous health and environmental benefits, the plant-based revolution also presents a promising solution to the prevention of soil erosion and degradation. Traditionally, livestock farming has been a major contributor to the loss of topsoil and degradation of fertile land. The intensive grazing and trampling by livestock can lead to compaction of the soil, making it more vulnerable to erosion by wind and water. The overuse of chemical fertilizers and pesticides in conventional agriculture practices further exacerbates soil degradation. By shifting towards a plant-based diet, we can significantly reduce the demand for livestock farming and the subsequent negative impacts on soil health. Instead, plant-based diets emphasize the cultivation of a diverse range of crops, which can help promote soil health and prevent erosion. The cultivation of legumes, for example, can increase soil nitrogen levels naturally, reducing the need for synthetic fertilizers. By employing practices like crop rotation and cover cropping, we can enhance soil structure and prevent erosion, ultimately leading to improved long-term soil productivity and agricultural sustainability.

THE ROLE OF PLANT-BASED DIETS IN ENERGY CONSERVATION

As the global demand for food continues to rise, the pressure to find sustainable and efficient food production methods becomes increasingly important. One solution lies in the adoption of plant-based diets, which have been proven to play a significant role in energy conservation. Plant-based diets primarily rely on the consumption of fruits, vegetables, legumes, and grains, which require substantially fewer resources compared to animal farming. Plants directly convert sunlight into energy through photosynthesis, bypassing the inefficient process of converting plant biomass into animal protein. By consuming plants directly, we can reduce the energy loss that occurs at every trophic level in the food chain. Plant-based diets have a significantly smaller carbon footprint compared to animal-based diets. Livestock production is one of the largest contributors to greenhouse gas emissions, deforestation, and water pollution. By shifting towards plant-based diets, we can mitigate the negative environmental impacts associated with animal agriculture, conserving energy and promoting a more sustainable future for our planet.

ENERGY REQUIREMENTS FOR PLANT-BASED FOOD PRODUCTION

One of the key aspects of the plant-based revolution is its focus on environmental sustainability. A major driver of this sustainability is the reduced energy requirements for plant-based food production compared to traditional livestock farming. Plant-based farming can significantly reduce the energy consumption associated with food production due to several factors. Firstly, plants require less energy input to grow compared to animals. This is because plants can convert sunlight into energy through photosynthesis, while animals need to eat plants to obtain energy, resulting in energy loss at each trophic level. The production of plant-based foods requires less energy-intensive activities such as transportation and processing compared to animal-based products. The transportation of plant-based foods often requires fewer refrigeration and storage needs, reducing energy consumption. Plant-based agriculture practices such as crop rotation and organic farming can further mitigate energy requirements by reducing the need for synthetic fertilizers and pesticides. The energy requirements for plant-based food production are significantly lower, making it a more sustainable option for feeding a growing global population.

THE POTENTIAL FOR RENEWABLE ENERGY IN THE PLANT-BASED SECTOR

As the world's population continues to grow, so does the demand for food and energy. The current reliance on fossil fuels and non-renewable resources is neither sustainable nor environmentally friendly. The plant-based sector offers a promising solution to this dilemma. Plant-based products, such as biofuels and biomass, can be used to generate renewable energy. Biofuels, derived from crops like corn, sugarcane, or soybeans, can be used to replace traditional fossil fuels in transportation. They offer a cleaner, more sustainable alternative that reduces greenhouse gas emissions and dependence on finite resources. Biomass, which includes organic waste and plant materials, can be converted into bioenergy through processes like anaerobic digestion or combustion. This renewable energy source can be used for heating, electricity generation, or even as a feedstock for the production of biofuels. By harnessing the power of plants, the plant-based sector has the potential to revolutionize the energy industry and pave the way towards a more sustainable future.

REDUCING THE ENERGY FOOTPRINT OF THE FOOD INDUSTRY

The food industry is notorious for its high energy consumption, from the production and processing of crops to the transportation and storage of food products. One effective solution to mitigate the energy footprint of the food industry is to encourage the adoption of plant-based diets. Plant-based diets predominantly rely on the consumption of fruits, vegetables, legumes, nuts, and seeds, which require significantly less energy to produce compared to animal-based products. By reducing the demand for animal agriculture, plant-based diets contribute to the reduction of greenhouse gas emissions associated with the livestock industry. The food industry should strive to optimize energy use throughout the entire food supply chain by implementing sustainable practices such as energy-efficient processing and packaging systems, as well as investing in renewable energy sources. By prioritizing energy reduction in the food industry, we can make substantial progress towards a more sustainable and environmentally friendly future.

THE ROLE OF PLANT-BASED DIETS IN AIR QUALITY

The link between food production and environmental impact has gained increasing attention. One area that has received considerable focus is the role of plant-based diets in improving air quality. Industrial livestock farming, a major contributor to greenhouse gas emissions and air pollution, releases large quantities of methane and nitrogen oxides into the atmosphere. These pollutants not only contribute to global warming but also lead to the formation of smog and respiratory problems. On the other hand, plant-based diets have been shown to have a significantly lower carbon footprint and emit fewer air pollutants. A study conducted by the University of Oxford found that switching to plant-based diets could reduce global greenhouse gas emissions by up to 70%. Consuming a plant-based diet reduces the demand for animal agriculture, thereby decreasing deforestation rates and the release of pollutants associated with land-use change. Promoting plant-based diets can play a crucial role in mitigating air pollution and promoting healthier environments.

THE REDUCTION OF GREENHOUSE GASES FROM PLANT-BASED DIETS

The production of animal-based products such as meat and dairy is one of the leading contributors to greenhouse gas emissions. Livestock production leads to the release of methane, a potent greenhouse gas that has a much higher heat trapping capability than carbon dioxide. The production and transportation of animal feed require considerable resources, including land, water, and energy. By shifting towards plant-based diets, individuals can significantly reduce their carbon footprint. Plants have a much lower greenhouse gas emission profile compared to animal products. The cultivation of plants for consumption requires fewer resources, making it a more sustainable choice. Plant-based diets also have the potential to mitigate other environmental issues, such as deforestation and water pollution, as they do not contribute to the expansion of agricultural land to meet the increasing demand for animal products. The adoption of plant-based diets can play a critical role in reducing greenhouse gas emissions and promoting a more sustainable future.

THE IMPACT ON AIR POLLUTION AND PUBLIC HEALTH

Animal agriculture, a major contributor to greenhouse gas emissions, is responsible for releasing large quantities of pollutants into the atmosphere. These pollutants, including ammonia, methane, and nitrous oxide, can have detrimental effects on air quality and contribute to the formation of smog and harmful particulate matter. By adopting a plant-based diet, individuals can significantly reduce their carbon footprint and help mitigate the adverse impacts of air pollution on public health. The production and consumption of animal-based foods have been linked to various health issues. High intake of animal products has been associated with an increased risk of chronic diseases, such as heart disease, stroke, and certain types of cancers. On the other hand, a plant-based diet rich in fruits, vegetables, whole grains, and legumes provides essential nutrients, antioxidants, and fiber that can support optimal health and prevent the onset of these diseases. Reducing the demand for animal products can alleviate the negative environmental and health impacts associated with intensive animal farming practices, including antibiotic resistance and the release of pollutants into water bodies. Thus, the plant-based revolution offers a promising pathway towards improving both air quality and public health.

THE ROLE OF DIET IN MITIGATING CLIMATE CHANGE

According to recent research, the role of diet in mitigating climate change is of utmost importance. The current food system heavily relies on animal agriculture, which contributes significantly to greenhouse gas emissions, deforestation, and water pollution. A shift towards a plant-based diet can significantly reduce these negative impacts on the environment. Plant-based diets have been found to require fewer resources and generate lower greenhouse gas emissions compared to animal-based diets. This is mainly because plants require fewer land, water, and feed inputs to produce food. The production of plant-based foods has the potential to restore degraded lands and promote biodiversity. Adopting a plant-based diet can have positive co-benefits, such as improving public health and reducing healthcare costs. The increased consumption of fruits, vegetables, whole grains, and legumes can lead to a lower risk of chronic diseases, including cardiovascular diseases and certain types of cancer. The promotion of a plant-based diet is crucial in tackling climate change and improving human health simultaneously. It requires a significant shift in consumer behavior, policy changes, and investment in sustainable agriculture practices.

THE ROLE OF PLANT-BASED DIETS IN WILDLIFE PROTECTION

The global demand for animal products has surged, leading to intensified industrial farming practices that wreak havoc on the environment and pose significant threats to wildlife populations. The adoption of plant-based diets has emerged as a viable solution to address these challenges and protect wildlife. By shifting away from animal agriculture and opting for plant-based alternatives, individuals can reduce their carbon footprint, minimize deforestation, and conserve critical habitats that are under constant threat. Plant-based diets also diminish the need for land to be cleared for livestock grazing and the production of animal feed, thereby curbing greenhouse gas emissions and safeguarding biodiversity. The decrease in animal farming supports the preservation of endangered species by mitigating wildlife trafficking, as demand for their body parts and products decrease. Plant-based diets promote the sustainable use of resources, ensuring that future generations will be able to coexist harmoniously with a wide range of wildlife. The adoption of plant-based diets plays a pivotal role in wildlife protection and is an essential step towards a more sustainable and ecologically responsible future.

HABITAT PRESERVATION THROUGH REDUCED ANIMAL FARMING

One effective method of habitat preservation is through the reduction of animal farming. Animal agriculture is a major driver of deforestation, habitat destruction, and biodiversity loss. The expansion of animal farming requires large-scale land clearance for grazing and growing animal feed crops, resulting in the destruction of natural habitats. The production of animal feed often involves the use of harmful chemicals, such as fertilizers and pesticides, which further degrade ecosystems and disrupt the balance of natural habitats. By transitioning to plant-based diets and reducing our dependency on animal products, we can significantly decrease the demand for animal farming and alleviate its negative impacts on habitat preservation. Plant-based diets not only require less land and water resources but also generate lower greenhouse gas emissions compared to animal-based diets. This shift in dietary choices can greatly contribute to the protection of natural habitats, allowing ecosystems to recover and wildlife populations to thrive. Promoting sustainable farming practices and supporting local organic agriculture are also important strategies to reduce the ecological footprint of our food systems and preserve habitats for future generations.

THE IMPACT ON ENDANGERED SPECIES

The current global food system heavily relies on animal agriculture, which has led to habitat destruction and loss of biodiversity. As a result, many species are on the brink of extinction. The transition to a plant-based diet can significantly mitigate this issue. By shifting away from animal agriculture, we can reduce the demand for land, water, and resources needed to raise livestock. This, in turn, would reduce deforestation and protect the natural habitats of endangered species. Plant-based diets have lower greenhouse gas emissions compared to animal-based diets. This is critical as climate change is one of the primary drivers of biodiversity loss. By curbing our contribution to climate change through the adoption of plant-based diets, we can help preserve the habitats and ecosystems that endangered species rely on. The plant-based revolution offers a sustainable and ethical solution to the pressing issue of endangered species, ensuring their survival and maintaining the delicate balance of our planet's ecosystems.

BIODIVERSITY BENEFITS OF PLANT-BASED EATING

Plant-based diets, which primarily consist of fruits, vegetables, legumes, whole grains, and nuts, have the potential to reduce the negative impact of food production on biodiversity. The agricultural industry is a significant driver of deforestation, habitat destruction, and species extinction due to the vast amount of land required for animal livestock and feed production. By shifting towards plant-based eating, demand for animal products would decrease, leading to a reduction in land use for livestock farming and the subsequent restoration of natural habitats. Plant-based diets often emphasize organic and locally sourced produce, which can reduce the reliance on monocultures, pesticide use, and transportation emissions that harm biodiversity. The cultivation of plants for direct human consumption requires less water, fertilizer, and energy compared to animal agriculture, further mitigating the negative impact on ecosystems. Thus, embracing plant-based diets is not only beneficial for personal health but also crucial for promoting and preserving biodiversity for future generations.

THE ROLE OF PLANT-BASED DIETS IN COMMUNITY BUILDING

In today's society, the role of plant-based diets goes beyond individual health benefits and extends into community building. Plant-based diets promote inclusivity and social cohesion by bridging cultural divides and fostering shared values. By adopting a plant-based lifestyle, individuals can connect with others who share their dietary preferences, creating a sense of community and belonging. Plant-based diets have the potential to break down barriers between different cultural and ethnic groups. Vegan and vegetarian restaurants often incorporate diverse flavors and ingredients from various cuisines, attracting customers from different backgrounds. This cross-cultural exchange at the dining table not only promotes tolerance and understanding but also encourages dialogue and collaboration among communities. The environmental sustainability associated with plant-based diets often becomes a rallying point for communities interested in combating climate change. By advocating for plant-based diets collectively, communities can strive towards a shared goal of creating a healthier and more sustainable future. Plant-based diets have the power to transcend individual choices and become a catalyst for community building on multiple levels.

PLANT-BASED EVENTS AND SOCIAL GATHERINGS

These events serve as platforms for individuals to come together and celebrate their commitment to a healthier and more sustainable way of living. One such event is the annual "Vegan Food Festival", where attendees can indulge in a wide variety of plant-based delicacies, attend cooking demonstrations, and learn about the environmental and ethical impacts of their food choices. These events not only provide education and awareness but also create a sense of community among like-minded individuals. Plant-based social gatherings such as potlucks and dinner parties offer opportunities for friends and families to share delicious and nutritious meals while expanding their culinary horizons. Such events encourage people to experiment with plant-based recipes and discover new flavors, ultimately promoting a shift towards a more plant-centered diet. As the plant-based movement continues to grow, these events and gatherings play a vital role in connecting people, fostering a sense of belonging, and inspiring others to join the plant-based revolution.

SUPPORT GROUPS AND NETWORKS FOR PLANT-BASED LIVING

Support groups and networks play a crucial role in fostering plant-based living and its positive impacts. These groups provide individuals with a platform to connect, share experiences, and seek advice, which can be particularly beneficial for those transitioning to a plant-based lifestyle. By engaging in conversations and interacting with like-minded individuals, participants can enhance their knowledge about plant-based eating, learn new recipes, and gain insights into the challenges and successes associated with this lifestyle choice. Support groups and networks can serve as a source of motivation and encouragement, especially during difficult times or when faced with criticism from others. The shared sense of community strengthens individuals' commitment to plant-based living, enabling them to overcome obstacles and stay true to their values. These networks often organize events, workshops, and educational sessions that facilitate personal growth and enable individuals to actively contribute to the plant-based movement. By providing a supportive and inclusive space, support groups and networks are instrumental in promoting plant-based living among individuals seeking healthier, more sustainable, and compassionate lifestyles.

THE CREATION OF INCLUSIVE AND DIVERSE COMMUNITIES

In the context of the plant-based revolution, this concept becomes even more significant as it invites individuals from various backgrounds to join a movement that is centered on the well-being of animals, human health, and the environment. By actively encouraging inclusivity and diversity within plant-based communities, we can bridge gaps between different cultures, religions, and socioeconomic classes. This emphasis on inclusivity not only broadens the reach of the movement but also allows for the exchange of ideas and experiences, enriching the collective knowledge and understanding of all involved. By recognizing and valuing the perspectives of individuals from different walks of life, we can create a space where everyone feels heard and respected. Embracing diversity within plant-based communities can also help to dispel the misconception that veganism is exclusive or inaccessible to certain groups. Through open dialogue, education, and outreach initiatives, we can work towards building inclusive and diverse communities that promote a more sustainable and compassionate future for all.

THE ROLE OF PLANT-BASED DIETS IN PERSONAL WELL-BEING

Plant-based diets have gained significant attention in recent years for their potential to improve personal well-being. XLVIII. Numerous studies have shown that following a plant-based diet can lower the risk of chronic diseases such as heart disease, diabetes, and certain types of cancer. These diets are typically rich in fruits, vegetables, whole grains, legumes, and nuts, which provide an abundance of essential vitamins, minerals, and fiber. By consuming an array of plant-based foods, individuals can ensure a diverse nutrient intake that supports optimal physiological function. Plant-based diets tend to be lower in saturated fats and cholesterol while being higher in dietary fiber, which can contribute to improved weight management and lower cholesterol levels. Research suggests that adherence to a plant-based diet may promote mental health and well-being. The inclusion of nutrient-dense foods and the absence of processed meats and high-fat dairy products may positively impact mood and cognitive function. Embracing a plant-based diet can play a significant role in enhancing personal well-being and overall health.

MENTAL HEALTH BENEFITS OF PLANT-BASED EATING

Studies have shown that individuals who follow a plant-based diet experience lower rates of depression and anxiety compared to those who consume more animal products. This may be attributed to the higher intake of nutrients found in plant-based foods, such as fiber, antioxidants, and phytochemicals, which have been shown to support brain health and reduce inflammation. Plant-based diets tend to be lower in saturated fats and cholesterol, which have been linked to an increased risk of mental health disorders. The consumption of plant-based foods has been associated with improved gut health and increased diversity of gut microbiota, which is known to play a crucial role in mood regulation. Plant-based diets also promote mindfulness and a sense of connection to nature, both of which can positively impact mental well-being. Adopting a plant-based eating pattern can be a powerful tool in promoting mental health and well-being.

THE CONNECTION BETWEEN DIET AND EMOTIONAL HEALTH

Studies have shown that there is a strong correlation between what we eat and our emotional well-being. A diet rich in whole foods, such as fruits, vegetables, and whole grains, has been associated with lower levels of depression and anxiety. On the other hand, a diet high in processed foods and sugar has been linked to an increased risk of mental health disorders. This connection can be attributed to several factors. For one, the nutrients found in whole foods, such as omega-3 fatty acids and antioxidants, have been shown to have a positive impact on brain health. A diet high in processed foods can lead to inflammation in the body, which has been linked to depression and other mood disorders. The gut-brain axis, the bidirectional communication system between the gut and the brain, plays a crucial role in emotional regulation. The bacteria in our gut, influenced by our diet, produce neurotransmitters that have a direct impact on our mood. It is evident that our diet choices can significantly impact our emotional well-being.

LIFESTYLE SATISFACTION AMONG PLANT-BASED DIETERS

As more individuals adopt plant-based diets, researchers and health professionals are curious about the impact on their overall satisfaction with life. Studies have suggested a positive association between consuming a plant-based diet and higher levels of life satisfaction. One reason for this might be the improved physical health outcomes often observed in plant-based dieters, such as lower body mass index and reduced risk of chronic diseases. These improved health outcomes can lead to greater overall well-being and satisfaction. Plant-based diets are often associated with ethical beliefs, such as reducing harm to animals and promoting environmental sustainability. Adhering to these values may provide a sense of purpose and contribute to an individual's overall contentment. Plant-based diets often involve consuming a variety of fruits, vegetables, whole grains, and legumes, which are rich in essential nutrients and phytochemicals that have been linked to improved mental health outcomes, including decreased risk of depression and anxiety. Thus, the adoption of a plant-based diet may contribute to increased lifestyle satisfaction among individuals who prioritize their health, ethical beliefs, and overall well-being.

THE ROLE OF PLANT-BASED DIETS IN LIFE-LONG HEALTH

There has been a notable shift in dietary choices towards plant-based diets. Plant-based diets primarily consist of fruits, vegetables, grains, legumes, and nuts, while minimizing or eliminating animal products. The increasing popularity of these diets can be attributed to the growing awareness of the numerous health benefits they offer. Research has consistently shown that plant-based diets are associated with a reduced risk of chronic diseases, including obesity, type 2 diabetes, heart disease, and certain types of cancer. Plant-based diets have been found to promote weight loss, improve blood glucose control, lower blood pressure, and reduce cholesterol levels. These positive outcomes are likely due to the high fiber content and rich array of phytochemicals present in plant-based foods. The absence of saturated and trans fats, commonly found in animal products, further contributes to the health-promoting effects of plant-based diets. Considering the substantial evidence supporting the benefits of plant-based diets, it is clear that adopting a plant-based lifestyle can significantly contribute to life-long health and well-being.

LONGEVITY AND PLANT-BASED DIETARY PATTERNS

Evidence suggests that individuals who follow plant-based diets tend to have a lower risk of developing chronic diseases such as cardiovascular disease, type 2 diabetes, and certain types of cancer, all of which are major causes of mortality. The inclusion of a higher proportion of plant-based food sources, such as fruits, vegetables, whole grains, legumes, nuts, and seeds, provides a wide range of essential nutrients, including fiber, vitamins, minerals, and phytochemicals. These components have been associated with numerous health benefits, including reduced inflammation, improved blood lipid profiles, and enhanced gut health. Plant-based diets are typically lower in saturated fat and cholesterol, while being higher in antioxidants and other bioactive compounds, which may contribute to lower rates of age-related diseases and overall mortality. The consumption of plant-based diets has been shown to promote greater weight loss and weight management, leading to a reduced risk of obesity-related illnesses. Thus, incorporating plant-based dietary patterns into one's lifestyle may have significant implications for promoting longevity and fostering a healthier population.

THE ROLE OF DIET IN HEALTHY AGING

As individuals enter their later years, proper nutrition becomes increasingly essential in maintaining overall health and preventing the onset of chronic diseases. A plant-based diet has been shown to be particularly beneficial in promoting healthy aging. Research indicates that individuals who consume a predominantly plant-based diet, rich in fruits, vegetables, whole grains, and legumes, experience a reduced risk of developing age-related health conditions such as cardiovascular disease, type 2 diabetes, and certain types of cancer. The abundance of antioxidants, vitamins, minerals, and fiber found in plant-based foods contribute to improved immune function, reduced inflammation, and enhanced cognitive function. This type of diet is typically lower in saturated fat and cholesterol, making it ideal for maintaining healthy cholesterol levels and promoting heart health. Plant-based diets have been associated with a healthy body weight, which in turn reduces the risk of obesity-related diseases. By adopting a plant-based diet, individuals can positively impact their long-term health and foster a better quality of life as they age.

PREVENTING AGE-RELATED DISEASES WITH PLANT-BASED NUTRITION

Research suggests that adopting a plant-based diet can potentially reduce the risk of chronic diseases commonly associated with aging. Plant-based foods are rich in essential nutrients such as vitamins, minerals, and antioxidants that play a crucial role in maintaining overall health and preventing age-related ailments. The consumption of fruits, vegetables, whole grains, legumes, and nuts has been linked to lower rates of heart disease, stroke, type 2 diabetes, and certain types of cancer. Plant-based diets are typically low in saturated fat and cholesterol, which can contribute to the development of cardiovascular diseases. The high fiber content found in plant-based foods helps regulate digestion, control blood sugar levels, and promote weight management, reducing the risk of obesity and related complications. Incorporating plant-based nutrition into one's diet can be a proactive approach to prevent age-related diseases and promote healthy aging.

THE ROLE OF PLANT-BASED DIETS IN CHILDREN'S HEALTH

One crucial aspect of the plant-based revolution lies in its potential to greatly impact children's health. With the rise in childhood obesity and chronic diseases such as diabetes, there is an urgent need for dietary interventions that prioritize nutrient-dense, plant-based foods. Numerous studies have shown that plant-based diets can improve children's overall health and reduce the risk of developing these chronic diseases. Plant-based diets are typically rich in fruits, vegetables, whole grains, legumes, and nuts, which provide essential vitamins, minerals, fiber, and antioxidants necessary for growth and development. Plant-based diets are naturally low in saturated fats and cholesterol, leading to a reduced risk of heart disease. Plant-based diets have been found to enhance gut microbiota composition, which plays a crucial role in immune system function and disease prevention. By promoting the consumption of plant-based diets in children, both the short-term and long-term health outcomes can be improved, helping to cultivate a generation of healthier individuals.

NUTRITIONAL ADEQUACY FOR GROWING BODIES

As children and adolescents undergo rapid growth and development, they require optimal nutrition to support their physical and cognitive development. Some critics argue that plant-based diets may be deficient in essential nutrients such as protein, calcium, iron, and vitamin B12, which are typically abundant in animal-based foods. With proper planning and education, a well-balanced and diverse plant-based diet can provide all the necessary nutrients for growing bodies. Plant-based sources such as legumes, tofu, seeds, nuts, whole grains, and leafy greens can offer ample amounts of protein, calcium, iron, and other essential nutrients. Fortified plant-based milks, cereals, and supplements can fulfill the requirements for vitamin B12, which is predominantly found in animal-based products. It is imperative that individuals, especially parents and caregivers, consult with registered dietitians or healthcare professionals to ensure adequate nutrient intake and monitor growth parameters in children following a plant-based diet. By addressing these concerns and taking appropriate measures, a plant-based diet can meet the nutritional needs of growing bodies, promoting long-term health and sustainability.

PLANT-BASED DIETS IN SCHOOLS AND EDUCATIONAL SETTINGS

Plant-based diets are becoming increasingly popular in schools and educational settings as a means of promoting healthier eating habits and environmental sustainability. Given the growing concern over childhood obesity and the impact of animal agriculture on the environment, many schools are adopting plant-based menus and incorporating educational programs on the benefits of these diets. Plant-based diets emphasize the consumption of fruits, vegetables, whole grains, legumes, and nuts, while minimizing or eliminating animal products. Numerous studies have shown that plant-based diets can help reduce the risk of chronic diseases, including heart disease, diabetes, and certain cancers. These diets are lower in saturated fats and cholesterol while being rich in fiber, vitamins, minerals, and phytochemicals, which are all essential for optimal health and well-being. By introducing plant-based diets in schools, students can develop healthier eating patterns, improve their overall health, and gain a better understanding of the environmental impact of food choices. Consequently, incorporating plant-based diets in educational settings has the potential to foster a generation of individuals who are conscious of their dietary choices and committed to promoting a sustainable and healthy future.

FOSTERING HEALTHY EATING HABITS FROM A YOUNG AGE

The adoption of plant-based diets has gained attention as a promising approach to achieving these goals. Introducing children to a diet centered around fruits, vegetables, whole grains, and legumes can provide numerous health benefits. Such a diet is rich in essential nutrients, vitamins, and minerals necessary for growth and development. The consumption of plant-based foods can help prevent obesity, heart disease, type 2 diabetes, and certain forms of cancer. By instilling healthy eating habits early on, parents and educators can equip children with the skills and knowledge necessary to make informed food choices throughout their lives. Schools and communities play a pivotal role in this process, offering opportunities for nutrition education and promoting access to healthy food options. Encouraging children to participate in growing and cooking their own food can also enhance their appreciation for plant-based meals and empower them to make healthier choices independently. Fostering healthy eating habits from a young age is vital for cultivating a generation that values and prioritizes their health and well-being.

THE ROLE OF PLANT-BASED DIETS IN WOMEN'S HEALTH

One significant aspect of the plant-based revolution is the role of plant-based diets in women's health. Numerous studies have highlighted the benefits of consuming a predominantly plant-based diet for women, particularly in relation to various health conditions. Research suggests that plant-based diets can significantly reduce the risk of developing chronic diseases, such as heart disease, diabetes, and certain types of cancer, which are major concerns for women's health. Plant-based diets have been found to support hormonal balance in women. By incorporating a variety of fruits, vegetables, whole grains, legumes, and nuts, women can ensure they receive an adequate intake of essential nutrients that play a crucial role in regulating hormonal function. Plant-based diets have also been associated with better menstrual health outcomes, including reduced menstrual pain and a lower risk of developing menstrual disorders. By adopting a plant-based diet, women can potentially improve their overall health and well-being, highlighting the significant impact of plant-based diets on women's health in the context of the plant-based revolution.

ADDRESSING SPECIFIC NUTRITIONAL NEEDS

While a plant-based diet is generally associated with several health benefits, it is crucial to ensure that individuals meet their specific nutritional requirements. One particular need that must be addressed is protein intake. Many people erroneously assume that plant-based diets are deficient in protein. Numerous plant-based sources such as legumes, tofu, tempeh, and quinoa are rich in protein content, providing ample opportunities to meet protein needs. Individuals following a plant-based diet need to pay attention to their intake of essential fatty acids, particularly omega-3 fatty acids, as they play a vital role in maintaining cardiovascular health and reducing inflammation. Sources of omega-3 fatty acids include chia seeds, flaxseeds, walnuts, and algae-based supplements. Individuals need to ensure adequate intake of vitamins and minerals such as calcium, iron, vitamin B12, and vitamin D. This can be achieved by incorporating foods such as leafy greens, almonds, lentils, fortified plant-based milks, and nutritional yeast into their diets. By addressing these specific nutritional needs, individuals can optimize their health and well-being while adopting a plant-based lifestyle.

THE IMPACT ON REPRODUCTIVE HEALTH

Studies have found that a diet rich in plant-based foods can positively influence reproductive health in both men and women. For women, consuming a variety of fruits, vegetables, whole grains, and legumes has been associated with a reduced risk of infertility, as well as improved overall reproductive function. This can be attributed to the higher intake of antioxidants, phyto-chemicals, and fiber found in plant-based foods, which help regulate hormonal balance, improve ovulation, and enhance the quality of eggs. In men, adopting a plant-based diet has shown benefits for sperm quality, with higher consumption of plant-based foods associated with higher sperm counts, motility, and morphology. Plant-based diets have been found to reduce the risk of certain reproductive health conditions, such as polycystic ovary syndrome (PCOS) and endometriosis, which can negatively impact fertility. The plant-based revolution offers promising avenues for optimizing reproductive health through dietary choices.

PLANT-BASED DIETS DURING PREGNANCY AND LACTATION

During pregnancy and lactation, it is crucial to pay attention to the nutritional needs of both the mother and the developing fetus or infant. Plant-based diets, which emphasize the consumption of fruits, vegetables, whole grains, legumes, nuts, and seeds, have gained popularity in recent years due to their numerous health benefits. There is limited research specifically focusing on the effects of plant-based diets during pregnancy and lactation. It is well-established that consuming a variety of plant-based foods can provide essential nutrients such as fiber, vitamins, minerals, and antioxidants. Adequate intake of these nutrients is crucial for maternal health and infant growth and development. Some studies have suggested that pregnant women following a plant-based diet may have a lower risk of gestational diabetes and high blood pressure. It is important for pregnant and lactating women following a plant-based diet to ensure proper intake of protein, iron, calcium, omega-3 fatty acids, and vitamin B12. Close monitoring by healthcare professionals, along with appropriate supplementation if required, is necessary to ensure both maternal and fetal health. Further research is needed to establish the long-term effects of plant-based diets during pregnancy and lactation, and to provide evidence-based guidelines for optimal nutrition in these critical periods.

THE ROLE OF PLANT-BASED DIETS IN MEN'S HEALTH

Plant-based diets have been gaining popularity in recent years, and their potential role in improving men's health should not be overlooked. Men's health concerns, such as heart disease, prostate cancer, and erectile dysfunction, can often be attributed to poor lifestyle choices and unhealthy diets. Research indicates that a plant-based diet can provide significant benefits in these areas. Plant-based diets are rich in fiber, vitamins, minerals, and antioxidants, which all contribute to better cardiovascular health. Studies have shown an association between plant-based diets and a reduced risk of prostate cancer. The inclusion of foods such as fruits, vegetables, legumes, and whole grains in a plant-based diet can also improve erectile function by promoting healthy blood flow. Plant-based diets have been linked to lower rates of obesity and type 2 diabetes, conditions that can greatly affect men's health. Despite these potential benefits, it is important to ensure that a plant-based diet is properly balanced and includes adequate protein, iron, and other essential nutrients to meet the unique nutritional needs of men.

ADDRESSING HEALTH CONCERNS SPECIFIC TO MEN

One such concern is prostate cancer, which is the most common cancer among men worldwide. Research has shown that a diet rich in fruits, vegetables, and whole grains can lower the risk of prostate cancer. Embracing a plant-based diet can serve as a preventive measure against this disease. Men face unique challenges in the field of mental health. Depression and anxiety are often less recognized and diagnosed in males, leading to a higher rate of suicide. It has been found that consuming a diet high in fruits and vegetables is associated with a reduced risk of depression. Promoting a plant-based diet can help address this mental health concern among men. Men are more likely to suffer from cardiovascular disease, the leading cause of death worldwide. By adopting a plant-based diet, which can lower cholesterol and blood pressure, men can mitigate the risk factors associated with heart disease. Addressing health concerns specific to men through a plant-based approach can have significant positive implications on their overall well-being.

THE ROLE OF DIET IN PREVENTING COMMON MALE DISEASES

One of the most prominent diseases that can be prevented through a healthy diet is prostate cancer. Research has shown that a diet rich in fruits, vegetables, and whole grains can significantly reduce the risk of developing this type of cancer. A plant-based diet has been found to reduce the risk of heart disease, which is another common male health issue. This can be attributed to the fact that plant-based foods are generally low in saturated fats and cholesterol, which are known to contribute to heart disease. A healthy diet can also play a crucial role in preventing obesity, which is associated with a wide range of male diseases such as diabetes, hypertension, and certain cancers. By consuming a balanced diet that includes a variety of nutrient-dense foods, men can protect themselves against these common diseases and improve their overall health and well-being. Understanding the role of diet in preventing common male diseases and making conscious dietary choices is paramount for men's health promotion.

PLANT-BASED DIETS AND TESTOSTERONE LEVELS

Plant-based diets have been gaining popularity in recent years due to their potential health benefits, including lower risks of chronic diseases such as obesity and heart disease. Concerns have been raised regarding the impact of plant-based diets on testosterone levels, particularly among men. Testosterone is a hormone that plays a vital role in male sexual development and function, as well as overall health. Some studies have suggested that a plant-based diet may lower testosterone levels, which could potentially lead to a decrease in muscle mass, energy levels, and libido. The evidence regarding the effect of plant-based diets on testosterone levels is conflicting. While some studies have indeed found lower testosterone levels in men who follow a vegetarian or vegan diet, others have reported no significant difference compared to those who consume animal products. It is important to consider that numerous other factors, such as age, exercise levels, and overall dietary patterns, can also impact testosterone levels. More research is needed to fully understand the relationship between plant-based diets and testosterone levels.

THE ROLE OF PLANT-BASED DIETS IN IMMUNE FUNCTION

Plant-based diets have gained considerable attention for their potential to improve immune function. Research suggests that a diet rich in plant-based foods, such as fruits, vegetables, whole grains, legumes, and nuts, can support a healthy immune system by providing essential nutrients and bioactive compounds. These nutrients include vitamins A, C, and E, as well as minerals like zinc and selenium, which are known to be vital for immune cell function and maintenance. Plant foods are abundant in antioxidants and phytochemicals, which have been shown to possess immune-boosting properties. Numerous studies have indicated that a plant-based diet can enhance immune responses, reduce inflammation, and prevent chronic diseases associated with impaired immune function, such as cardiovascular disease and certain types of cancer. Plant-based diets are typically low in saturated fat and high in fiber, leading to a healthy gut microbiome, which also plays a crucial role in immune system regulation. Adopting a plant-based diet can be a valuable strategy to support and optimize immune function, contributing to overall health and well-being.

BOOSTING IMMUNITY WITH PLANT-BASED NUTRIENTS

A plant-based diet rich in nutrients has been shown to have multiple benefits in boosting immunity. Many plant-based foods are packed with essential vitamins and minerals that play a crucial role in supporting immune function. Vitamin C, found in abundance in fruits such as oranges, strawberries, and kiwis, is known for its immune-boosting properties. Other plant-based nutrients like vitamin A, found in orange vegetables like carrots and sweet potatoes, play a key role in maintaining immune health as well. Plant-based foods are typically high in antioxidants, which can help protect the body against oxidative stress and inflammation, both of which can compromise immune function. A plant-based diet can contribute to a healthy gut microbiome, where the majority of our immune system resides. The fiber in plant-based foods acts as prebiotics, providing nourishment for beneficial gut bacteria, thus promoting a diverse and robust immune system. Incorporating plant-based nutrients into one's diet can be a powerful strategy in boosting immunity and maintaining optimal health.

THE ROLE OF ANTIOXIDANTS AND ANTI-INFLAMMATORY FOODS

Antioxidants are substances that help to protect the body against free radicals, which are harmful molecules that can damage cells and contribute to the development of chronic diseases such as cancer, heart disease, and diabetes. By neutralizing these free radicals, antioxidants can mitigate their adverse effects and support the body's natural defense mechanisms. Anti-inflammatory foods, on the other hand, help to reduce inflammation in the body. Chronic inflammation has been implicated in the pathogenesis of various diseases, including cardiovascular disease, obesity, and autoimmune disorders. By including foods rich in antioxidants, such as fruits, vegetables, nuts, and whole grains, as well as anti-inflammatory foods like fatty fish, olive oil, and turmeric, individuals can positively influence their health outcomes. Scientific evidence suggests that a plant-based diet, which inherently includes a variety of antioxidant and anti-inflammatory foods, may be particularly beneficial in preventing and managing chronic diseases.

DIETARY PATTERNS AND RESISTANCE TO ILLNESS

Dietary patterns play a crucial role in determining an individual's resistance to illness. A plant-based diet has been found to be particularly effective in promoting overall immune health and preventing various chronic diseases. A study conducted by McEvoy and colleagues (2019) revealed that individuals following a plant-based diet had higher levels of immune cells, such as natural killer cells and T cells, which are essential for fighting off infections and diseases. Plant-based diets are typically rich in antioxidants, vitamins, and minerals, which have been shown to boost the immune system and reduce inflammation. On the other hand, diets high in animal products, processed foods, and added sugars have been associated with increased inflammation and a weakened immune system. A plant-based diet contributes to maintaining a healthy gut microbiome, which is directly linked to immune function. The fibers and prebiotics found in plant-based foods help nourish the gut microbiota, promoting the growth of beneficial bacteria that enhance immune response. Adopting a plant-based dietary pattern can significantly contribute to one's resistance to illness and overall well-being.

THE ROLE OF PLANT-BASED DIETS IN COGNITIVE FUNCTION

A growing body of research has explored the role of plant-based diets in cognitive function. Studies have consistently shown that consuming a diet rich in plant-based foods, such as fruits, vegetables, whole grains, and legumes, is associated with improved cognitive performance. A study published in the Journal of the Academy of Nutrition and Dietetics found that adhering to a plant-based diet was associated with better memory, attention, and processing speed in older adults. This could be attributed to the abundance of nutrients found in plant-based foods, such as antioxidants, vitamins, and minerals, which are known to support brain health. Plant-based diets are also typically low in saturated fat and cholesterol, which have been linked to increased risk of cognitive decline and neurodegenerative diseases. The high fiber content of plant-based diets may contribute to improved cognitive function by promoting healthy gut microbiota, which have been found to play a crucial role in brain health. These findings highlight the potential benefits of plant-based diets in enhancing cognitive function and provide further support for the plant-based revolution.

THE IMPACT ON BRAIN HEALTH AND MENTAL CLARITY

Research indicates that consuming a plant-based diet can have positive effects on cognitive function and mental well-being. Plant-based foods, such as fruits, vegetables, nuts, and whole grains, are rich in antioxidants, vitamins, minerals, and phyto-chemicals essential for brain health. These nutrients have been shown to reduce inflammation, oxidative stress, and neuronal damage in the brain, thereby improving cognitive functions such as memory, attention, and learning abilities. A plant-based diet is associated with a reduced risk of developing mental health disorders, including depression and anxiety. A study conducted by the National Institutes of Health discovered that individuals who followed a plant-based diet had lower levels of mental distress compared to those who consumed a diet higher in animal products. The connection between plant-based eating and mental clarity can be attributed to the higher intake of nutrient-dense foods, which nourish the brain and promote overall well-being. Adopting a plant-based lifestyle can positively impact brain health and enhance mental clarity.

NUTRIENTS IMPORTANT FOR COGNITIVE DEVELOPMENT

One essential nutrient for cognitive development is omega-3 fatty acids. These fatty acids are primarily found in fatty fish, such as salmon and mackerel, as well as in certain plant-based sources like flaxseeds and walnuts. Omega-3 fatty acids are crucial for the development and maintenance of the brain, improving memory, attention, and overall cognitive performance. Another vital nutrient is iron, which is necessary for the synthesis and function of neurotransmitters in the brain. Iron deficiency can lead to impaired cognitive development, affecting attention, memory, and even IQ in severe cases. Good dietary sources of iron include lean meat, legumes, and dark leafy greens. Choline, an essential nutrient found in foods like eggs, poultry, and soybeans, is essential for the formation and maintenance of cell membranes in the brain. Choline also plays a significant role in the synthesis of neurotransmitters, which are vital for cognitive processes such as memory and learning. Ensuring adequate intake of these essential nutrients is crucial for optimal cognitive development.

THE POTENTIAL FOR PLANT-BASED DIETS TO PREVENT NEURODEGENERATIVE DISEASES

Evidence suggests that plant-based diets have the potential to prevent neurodegenerative diseases. Neurodegenerative diseases, such as Alzheimer's and Parkinson's, are characterized by the progressive loss of neurons in the brain. Several factors, including oxidative stress, chronic inflammation, and mitochondrial dysfunction, contribute to the development and progression of these diseases. Plant-based diets, rich in antioxidant and anti-inflammatory compounds, can mitigate these contributing factors and potentially prevent neurodegeneration. Phytochemicals present in a variety of plant foods, including fruits, vegetables, and whole grains, possess neuroprotective properties and can help combat oxidative stress. The anti-inflammatory effects of plant-based diets, due to the high intake of fiber and phytochemicals, can reduce chronic inflammation in the brain. Plant-based diets enhance mitochondrial function through the consumption of nutrient-dense foods that provide essential vitamins and minerals. Evidence from observational studies and clinical trials support the benefits of plant-based diets in reducing the risk and slowing the progression of neurodegenerative diseases. While further research is needed to fully understand the mechanisms behind these effects, current findings suggest that adopting a plant-based diet may be an effective preventative strategy against neurodegeneration.

THE ROLE OF PLANT-BASED DIETS IN DENTAL HEALTH

One important aspect of dental health that has gained attention in recent years is the role of plant-based diets. Research has shown that a diet rich in fruits, vegetables, nuts, and whole grains can have numerous benefits for oral health. Firstly, these types of foods are typically low in sugar, which is a major contributor to tooth decay. In contrast, a diet high in processed and sugary foods can lead to the production of acids that erode tooth enamel and increase the risk of cavities. Plant-based diets are often high in fiber, which can help promote good oral hygiene by stimulating saliva production and reducing the buildup of plaque. Many plant-based foods are rich in antioxidants and anti-inflammatory properties, which can help combat gum disease and reduce the risk of tooth loss. Incorporating more plant-based foods into one's diet can provide important benefits for dental health and contribute to overall oral well-being.

THE IMPACT OF DIET ON ORAL HYGIENE AND HEALTH

A diet rich in fruits, vegetables, and whole grains provides essential nutrients for maintaining optimal oral health. These foods are packed with vitamins and minerals, such as vitamin C, which helps strengthen the gums and promote gum health. The high fiber content of plant-based foods stimulates saliva production, aiding in the natural cleansing process of the mouth and reducing the risk of tooth decay. On the contrary, a diet high in sugar, processed foods, and acidic beverages can have detrimental effects on oral health. Excessive sugar consumption provides fuel for bacteria in the mouth, leading to the production of acids that erode tooth enamel and cause cavities. Similarly, acidic beverages like soda and sports drinks can weaken tooth enamel and contribute to the development of dental erosion. Adopting a plant-based diet and minimizing the intake of sugary and acidic foods and drinks can play a significant role in maintaining good oral hygiene and promoting overall health.

NUTRITIONAL CONSIDERATIONS FOR STRONG TEETH AND GUMS

Nutritional considerations play a crucial role in maintaining strong teeth and gums. A plant-based diet rich in essential nutrients can greatly contribute to oral health. Calcium, for instance, is imperative for the formation and development of strong teeth and bones. While dairy products are often associated with high calcium content, several plant-based sources such as kale, spinach, and almonds offer an equally substantial calcium supply. Alongside calcium, vitamin D is necessary for the body's proper absorption of this mineral. While limited dietary sources of plant-based vitamin D exist, exposure to sunlight can stimulate its synthesis in the skin. Vitamin C aids in collagen production, which is crucial for maintaining healthy gums. Citrus fruits, strawberries, and papaya are excellent plant-based sources of this vitamin. Polyphenols found in unsweetened green and black teas have been associated with the prevention of tooth decay by neutralizing harmful bacteria in the oral cavity. Thus, adopting a plant-based diet rich in calcium, vitamin D, vitamin C, and polyphenols can greatly contribute to promoting strong teeth and healthy gums.

THE RELATIONSHIP BETWEEN SUGAR CONSUMPTION AND PLANT-BASED EATING

As more people are transitioning to plant-based diets, it is essential to examine the impact of sugar consumption on overall health and wellness. Research indicates that excessive sugar intake is associated with various health issues, including obesity, type 2 diabetes, and cardiovascular diseases. Plant-based diets, on the other hand, have been shown to have numerous health benefits, such as lower body weight, improved blood glucose control, and reduced risk of chronic diseases. Since plant-based diets primarily consist of whole plant foods like fruits, vegetables, whole grains, and legumes, they naturally have lower levels of added sugars compared to the standard Western diet. By choosing plant-based foods, individuals can reduce their overall sugar intake and improve their health outcomes. It is crucial to note that not all plant-based foods are low in sugar, and added sugars can still be present in processed plant-based products. It is vital to make informed choices and opt for whole, unprocessed plant-based foods to maximize the benefits of a plant-based diet while minimizing excess sugar consumption.

THE ROLE OF PLANT-BASED DIETS IN SKIN HEALTH

There has been an increasing interest in the role of plant-based diets in skin health. LVI. Studies have shown that a diet rich in fruits, vegetables, and whole grains can have a positive impact on the overall health and appearance of the skin. The nutrients found in these foods, such as vitamins A, C, and E, as well as antioxidants, have been found to promote collagen production, protect against sun damage, and reduce inflammation. Plant-based diets are often lower in processed foods, which can contribute to skin issues such as acne and inflammation. Plant-based diets may also help to improve general skin conditions such as eczema, psoriasis, and rosacea. With the growing popularity of plant-based diets, more research is being conducted to explore the specific mechanisms by which these diets improve skin health. It is becoming increasingly clear that what we put into our bodies can have a significant impact on the health and appearance of our skin. Incorporating a plant-based diet into one's lifestyle may be an effective strategy for achieving optimal skin health.

THE BENEFITS OF A PLANT-BASED DIET FOR SKIN

A plant-based diet is not only beneficial for overall health but also for the skin. Research has shown that a diet rich in fruits, vegetables, whole grains, and plant-based proteins can promote a clear and youthful complexion. One of the main reasons behind this is the high antioxidant content of plant-based foods. Antioxidants help protect the skin by neutralizing harmful free radicals that can damage collagen and elastin fibers, leading to wrinkles and sagging skin. Plant-based foods are rich in vitamins and minerals that are essential for maintaining healthy skin. Vitamin C promotes collagen production and helps fight against skin inflammation, while vitamin E helps to moisturize the skin and protect it from oxidative stress. Plant-based diets are often lower in processed foods and animal fats, which have been linked to skin conditions like acne. By adopting a plant-based diet, individuals may experience fewer breakouts and a more radiant complexion.

NUTRIENTS THAT PROMOTE HEALTHY SKIN

In the pursuit of healthy skin, it is crucial to understand the role of nutrients in promoting its overall well-being. There are several key nutrients that have been found to effectively nourish the skin and enhance its health. Firstly, antioxidants play a vital role in preventing oxidative damage caused by free radicals in the environment. These compounds are commonly found in a variety of plant-based foods such as fruits, vegetables, and legumes. Omega-3 fatty acids possess anti-inflammatory properties that contribute to improving skin health by reducing redness and irritation. Foods rich in omega-3 fatty acids include flaxseeds, walnuts, and fatty fish like salmon. Vitamins A, C, and E are essential for maintaining healthy skin as they aid in collagen production, provide sun protection, and combat skin aging. These vitamins can be obtained from a range of plant-based sources like citrus fruits, leafy greens, and nuts. It is important to note that a balanced and diverse plant-based diet can provide the necessary nutrients to support healthy skin, leading to improved complexion and overall skin appearance.

THE IMPACT OF DAIRY AND MEAT ON SKIN CONDITIONS

Many studies have examined the effects of dairy and meat consumption on skin conditions, and a growing body of evidence suggests that these foods may exacerbate certain skin conditions. Dairy products, such as milk and cheese, have been implicated in conditions such as acne, eczema, and psoriasis. One proposed mechanism is the hormonal influence of dairy products, particularly the presence of hormones like insulin-like growth factor (IGF-1). These hormones can promote inflammation and increase sebum production, leading to acne breakouts. Meat consumption has also been associated with skin conditions. Some research suggests that the high levels of arachidonic acid found in meat may trigger inflammation and exacerbate conditions such as eczema. The excessive consumption of processed meats containing nitrites and preservatives may contribute to the development of certain skin conditions. These findings underscore the importance of considering the impact of diet on skin health and highlight the potential benefits of adopting a plant-based diet for individuals seeking to improve their skin conditions.

THE ROLE OF PLANT-BASED DIETS IN HORMONAL BALANCE

A growing body of research suggests that the consumption of plant-based foods can have a positive impact on hormonal regulation. A study conducted by Zhang et al. (2018) found that a plant-based diet rich in fruits, vegetables, whole grains, and legumes was associated with improved insulin sensitivity and lowered risk of insulin resistance. This is particularly significant because insulin plays a crucial role in hormone regulation, as it helps to control blood sugar levels and promote the production of other hormones. Plant-based diets have been linked to reduced levels of estrogen in the body, which may have important implications for both women and men. Elevated levels of estrogen in women have been associated with an increased risk of certain cancers, such as breast and ovarian cancer. In men, high estrogen levels have been linked to reduced testosterone production and may contribute to decreased fertility and sexual dysfunction. By consuming plant-based diets, individuals can potentially lower their estrogen levels and achieve a more balanced hormonal profile. The adoption of plant-based diets appears to offer a promising approach for achieving hormonal balance and promoting overall wellness. Further research is warranted to better understand the mechanisms through which plant-based diets exert their hormonal effects, as well as to explore the potential long-term benefits and risks associated with this dietary approach.

THE EFFECT OF DIET ON ENDOCRINE HEALTH

The endocrine system plays a crucial role in regulating various bodily functions, including metabolism, growth, and reproduction. Several studies have shown a clear link between diet and the function of the endocrine system. A diet high in processed foods and saturated fats has been associated with an increased risk of developing endocrine disorders such as obesity and type 2 diabetes. On the other hand, a plant-based diet rich in fruits, vegetables, whole grains, and legumes has been shown to have a positive impact on endocrine health. This dietary pattern is not only low in unhealthy fats but also high in fiber, vitamins, minerals, and antioxidants. These compounds have been shown to reduce inflammation, improve insulin sensitivity, and promote weight management, all of which are crucial for maintaining optimal endocrine function. Adopting a plant-based diet can be an effective strategy to support and enhance endocrine health.

PLANT-BASED FOODS THAT SUPPORT HORMONAL REGULATION

Plant-based foods have been shown to have numerous health benefits, including supporting hormonal regulation. One such plant-based food that is known to have a positive effect on hormonal balance is flaxseed. Flaxseed is rich in lignans, a type of phytoestrogen that has been found to help balance estrogen levels in the body. Phytoestrogens are natural compounds that have a similar structure to estrogen and can mimic its effects. Another plant-based food that supports hormonal regulation is soy. Soy contains isoflavones, which are also phytoestrogens that have been found to have estrogen-like effects in the body. These compounds can help regulate hormone levels and alleviate symptoms of hormonal imbalance. Cruciferous vegetables, such as broccoli and cauliflower, contain compounds called indoles that can support the metabolism of estrogen and aid in hormonal regulation. Incorporating plant-based foods into the diet can be beneficial for hormonal regulation and overall health.

THE IMPACT OF ANIMAL PRODUCTS ON HORMONE LEVELS

Animal products have been found to significantly impact hormone levels in the human body. Studies have shown that dairy products contain estrogen and progesterone, two hormones that can have noticeable effects on the endocrine system. Consuming these products can disrupt the balance of hormones in the body, leading to various health complications. The use of growth hormones and antibiotics in animal agriculture can also have negative effects on hormone levels. Growth hormones, such as those given to cows to increase milk production, can linger in animal products and be transferred to humans upon consumption. This can disrupt the delicate hormonal balance in the human body and contribute to the development of hormone-related diseases. The use of antibiotics in raising animals for food can affect hormone levels indirectly. Antibiotics can disrupt the gut microbiome, which plays a vital role in hormone regulation. Reducing or eliminating the consumption of animal products can be beneficial in maintaining optimal hormone levels and overall health.

THE ROLE OF PLANT-BASED DIETS IN ATHLETIC RECOVERY

Plant-based diets have been gaining popularity among athletes as a means to enhance recovery and optimize performance. Research suggests that these dietary choices can provide numerous benefits for athletes during the recovery process. Plant-based diets are rich in antioxidants which help reduce inflammation and oxidative stress caused by intense exercise. Plant proteins offer a complete amino acid profile necessary for muscle repair and rebuilding. The high fiber content in plant-based diets also plays a crucial role in promoting gut health, which is essential for proper nutrient absorption and immune function. The emphasis on whole foods in plant-based diets ensures adequate intake of essential vitamins, minerals, and phytonutrients necessary for tissue repair and overall wellbeing post-exercise. Several studies have shown that athletes following plant-based diets experience improved muscle glycogen replenishment, reduced muscle soreness, and enhanced immune function, leading to faster recovery and improved performance. These findings highlight the potential of plant-based diets as an effective tool for athletes seeking to optimize recovery and achieve their athletic goals.

NUTRITIONAL STRATEGIES FOR POST-EXERCISE RECOVERY

Adequate intake of essential macronutrients, such as carbohydrates and proteins, is essential during this recovery phase. Carbohydrates replenish glycogen stores, the body's main source of energy, while proteins aid in muscle protein synthesis, facilitating muscle repair and growth. Incorporating high-quality carbohydrates, such as whole grains and fruits, into post-workout meals can help restore glycogen levels efficiently. Consuming a protein-rich meal or supplement within the first hour after exercise can enhance muscle recovery by promoting the activation of muscle protein synthesis. Aside from macronutrients, micronutrients such as vitamins and minerals have shown to play a crucial role in post-exercise recovery. Vitamin C has been linked to reducing muscle soreness and inflammation, while minerals like magnesium and potassium are involved in muscle contractions and electrolyte balance. Ensuring an adequate intake of these essential micronutrients through a well-balanced diet or supplementation can further aid in the recovery process. Proper nutritional strategies post-exercise are fundamental for optimizing recovery, improving performance, and preventing excessive muscle damage.

ANTI-INFLAMMATORY EFFECTS OF PLANT-BASED FOODS

One of the most significant benefits of plant-based foods is their anti-inflammatory effects. Research shows that a diet rich in fruits, vegetables, whole grains, and legumes can reduce inflammation in the body. Inflammation is a natural response of the immune system to injury or infection, but chronic inflammation can lead to various diseases, including heart disease, diabetes, and certain types of cancer. Plant-based foods are filled with antioxidants and phytochemicals that have powerful anti-inflammatory properties. Fruits like berries and cherries contain anthocyanins, which can reduce inflammation and oxidative stress in the body. Vegetables such as leafy greens are packed with vitamins, minerals, and fiber that have been found to lower markers of inflammation. Whole grains like brown rice and quinoa contain compounds that can help regulate inflammation. Legumes, such as lentils and chickpeas, provide a good source of plant-based protein and also contain anti-inflammatory components. Incorporating a variety of plant-based foods into one's diet can help combat inflammation and promote overall good health.

THE ROLE OF PLANT-BASED PROTEIN IN MUSCLE REPAIR

Muscle repair is a vital process for individuals engaged in physical activities or athletes who undergo intense training. Protein plays a crucial role in this process, as it provides the necessary building blocks for muscle tissue regeneration. Traditionally, animal-based protein sources have been recommended for muscle repair due to their complete amino acid profile. Recent research has shown that plant-based protein can also effectively support muscle repair. In fact, plant-based proteins offer several advantages over their animal counterparts. Firstly, plant-based protein sources such as soy, quinoa, and hemp contain all nine essential amino acids required for muscle repair. These plant proteins also come with an array of beneficial phytochemicals and antioxidants that aid in reducing inflammation and oxidative stress, both of which can hinder muscle recovery. Plant-based protein sources are often lower in saturated fat, cholesterol, and overall energy content, thereby providing a healthful alternative for individuals looking to optimize muscle repair while simultaneously improving their overall health. The inclusion of plant-based protein in the diet can be an effective strategy for individuals seeking to support muscle repair and enhance recovery after physical exertion.

THE ROLE OF PLANT-BASED DIETS IN DIGESTIVE HEALTH

Plant-based diets have gained significant attention in recent years due to their potential role in promoting digestive health. Research has shown that these diets, primarily composed of fruits, vegetables, whole grains, legumes, and nuts, are rich in fiber, antioxidants, and phytochemicals, which are known to have beneficial effects on the gastrointestinal system. Fiber, in particular, plays a crucial role in maintaining a healthy digestive tract as it adds bulk to the stool and promotes regular bowel movements. The high content of antioxidants and phytochemicals found in plant-based diets can provide protection against inflammation and oxidative stress, which are associated with various digestive disorders such as irritable bowel syndrome and inflammatory bowel disease. The consumption of plant-based foods has been linked to a diverse gut microbiota, which is essential for proper digestion and nutrient absorption. Adopting a plant-based diet can contribute to improved digestive health by promoting bowel regularity, reducing inflammation, and supporting a healthy gut microbiota.

THE IMPORTANCE OF FIBER FOR GUT HEALTH

Fiber is a crucial component of a healthy diet as it plays a vital role in maintaining optimal gut function and overall well-being. Firstly, fiber aids in the regulation of bowel movements, preventing constipation and maintaining regularity. It adds bulk to the stool, allowing it to move through the digestive system smoothly. Secondly, fiber acts as a prebiotic, a type of food that promotes the growth and activity of beneficial gut bacteria. These bacteria help protect against harmful pathogens, strengthen the immune system, and enhance nutrient absorption. Fiber helps control blood sugar levels by slowing down the absorption of glucose into the bloodstream. This is especially beneficial for individuals with diabetes or insulin resistance. Consuming an adequate amount of fiber has been linked to a reduced risk of various chronic diseases, including cardiovascular disease, obesity, and certain types of cancer. Incorporating fiber-rich foods into one's diet is crucial for maintaining a healthy gut, promoting overall health, and preventing the onset of various illnesses.

PLANT-BASED DIETS AND THE MICROBIOME

Plant-based diets have gained significant attention due to their potential positive impact on the human microbiome. The microbiome refers to the trillions of microorganisms residing in and on our bodies, primarily in the gastrointestinal tract. Emerging research indicates that plant-based diets may promote a diverse and balanced microbiome composition, which is associated with various health benefits. Plant-based diets are typically rich in fiber, prebiotics, and polyphenols, all of which serve as fuel for the beneficial gut bacteria. These compounds are not easily digested by humans but can be fermented by the gut bacteria to produce short-chain fatty acids, such as butyrate, which possess numerous anti-inflammatory and protective properties. Plant-based diets have been found to reduce the abundance of potentially harmful bacteria, such as Firmicutes, while promoting the growth of beneficial bacteria, such as Bacteroidetes. Plant-based diets may enhance the production of protective mucus and support the gut barrier's integrity, further influencing the microbiome's health. As such, adopting a plant-based diet may significantly influence the composition and function of the microbiome, paving the way for improved overall health and disease prevention.

MANAGING DIGESTIVE DISORDERS WITH DIETARY CHANGES

Managing digestive disorders such as irritable bowel syndrome (IBS), Crohn's disease, and celiac disease can be challenging and debilitating for individuals. Recent research has shown promising results in managing these disorders through dietary changes. Adopting a plant-based diet, for instance, has been found to be beneficial due to its abundance of fiber, vitamins, and minerals. Fiber aids in regulating bowel movements and promoting healthy digestion, reducing the symptoms associated with IBS. A plant-based diet can be particularly beneficial for individuals with Crohn's disease, as it eliminates potential triggers such as dairy and gluten. Individuals with celiac disease can effectively manage their symptoms by eliminating gluten-containing foods from their diet. It is important to note, however, that each individual's needs may vary, and it is advisable to consult with a healthcare professional or registered dietitian before making any significant dietary changes. Nevertheless, dietary modifications offer a promising approach to managing digestive disorders and have the potential to greatly improve the quality of life for those affected by these conditions.

THE ROLE OF PLANT-BASED DIETS IN CARDIOVASCULAR HEALTH

Plant-based diets have gained significant attention in recent years for their potential to promote cardiovascular health. A growing body of evidence indicates that consumption of plant-based foods can reduce the risk of cardiovascular diseases such as heart disease and stroke. Several mechanisms underlie this protective effect. Firstly, plant-based diets are typically low in saturated fats and cholesterol, which are known contributors to the development of atherosclerosis and high blood pressure. Secondly, these diets are abundant in fiber, antioxidants, and phytochemicals, which have been shown to lower blood cholesterol levels, reduce inflammation, and improve endothelial function. The high intake of fruits, vegetables, and whole grains in plant-based diets provides an array of essential nutrients, including vitamins, minerals, and antioxidants, which collectively support cardiovascular health. Plant-based diets have been associated with weight loss and maintenance of healthy body weight, which further reduces the risk of cardiovascular diseases. Taken together, the body of evidence strongly suggests that plant-based diets play a crucial role in maintaining cardiovascular health and should be considered as part of a comprehensive approach to cardiovascular disease prevention and management.

THE IMPACT ON BLOOD PRESSURE AND CHOLESTEROL LEVELS

A study conducted by the Academy of Nutrition and Dietetics found that following a plant-based diet has a significant impact on blood pressure and cholesterol levels. Research has consistently shown that individuals who consume predominantly plant-based diets have lower blood pressure readings compared to those following a typically Western diet. This can be attributed to the low sodium content and high potassium levels found in plant-based foods, which help to maintain blood pressure within a healthy range. Plant-based diets have been shown to lower levels of LDL cholesterol, often referred to as the "bad" cholesterol. This is due to the absence of saturated fats found in animal products and the abundance of heart-healthy fats found in plant-based foods such as avocados, nuts, and seeds. Plant-based diets are rich in dietary fiber, which helps to reduce the absorption of cholesterol in the body. It is evident that adopting a plant-based diet can have a profound impact on blood pressure and cholesterol levels, making it an effective strategy for reducing the risk of cardiovascular diseases.

HEART-HEALTHY PLANT-BASED FOODS

Another key component of the plant-based revolution is the emphasis on heart-healthy plant-based foods. The consumption of these foods has been shown to have several positive effects on cardiovascular health. Studies have found that a diet rich in fruits and vegetables can lower the risk of heart disease. This is due to the high content of fiber, antioxidants, and phytochemicals found in these foods, which help reduce inflammation and improve blood vessel function. Plant-based diets tend to be low in saturated fats and cholesterol, both of which are known to contribute to heart disease. By replacing animal products with plant-based alternatives such as beans, legumes, and whole grains, individuals can lower their intake of these harmful substances and improve their heart health. Plant-based diets have been linked to lower blood pressure levels, a major risk factor for heart disease. Incorporating heart-healthy plant-based foods into one's diet can play a significant role in preventing and managing cardiovascular diseases, thus contributing to the overall health and well-being of individuals.

THE ROLE OF DIET IN PREVENTING HEART DISEASE

Numerous studies have shown that adopting a plant-based diet significantly reduces the risk of heart disease. Plant-based diets are rich in fruits, vegetables, whole grains, legumes, and nuts, which provide essential nutrients, vitamins, and minerals while considerably lowering the intake of saturated and trans fats. These types of fats are found primarily in animal-based products such as meat and dairy, and they have been strongly associated with an increased risk of heart disease. In contrast, plant-based diets are high in fiber and antioxidants, which help to lower cholesterol levels, reduce inflammation, and improve blood pressure. The consumption of plant-based proteins, such as beans and lentils, has also been linked to a decreased risk of heart disease. Studies have shown that incorporating plant sterols found in certain plant-based foods can help to lower LDL cholesterol levels. Adopting a plant-based diet can be an effective strategy to prevent heart disease and promote heart health.

THE ROLE OF PLANT-BASED DIETS IN CANCER PREVENTION

Plant-based diets have gained recognition for their potential role in the prevention of cancer. Various studies have shown that consuming a diet predominantly composed of plant-based foods can reduce the risk of developing certain types of cancer. The abundance of phytochemicals found in fruits, vegetables, and whole grains has been linked to their anti-carcinogenic properties. These compounds have been found to interfere with cancer cell growth, prevent DNA damage, and promote the elimination of potential carcinogens from the body. Plant-based diets are typically low in saturated fats and high in fiber, providing protective effects against cancer development. The intake of red and processed meats, on the other hand, has been associated with an increased risk of developing colorectal, prostate, and breast cancers. It is important to note that while plant-based diets can play a significant role in cancer prevention, they should be consumed as part of a balanced and varied diet to ensure adequate nutrient intake. Additional research is needed to fully understand the mechanisms behind the preventive effects of plant-based diets on cancer development.

DIETARY FACTORS IN CANCER RISK REDUCTION

Dietary factors play a crucial role in reducing the risk of cancer. Numerous studies have shown that a plant-based diet rich in fruits, vegetables, whole grains, and legumes can decrease the likelihood of developing various types of cancer. Fruits and vegetables, in particular, are abundant in antioxidants, vitamins, and minerals that help protect cells from damage caused by free radicals. These plant-based foods are high in fiber, which aids in maintaining a healthy weight and reducing the risk of obesity-related cancers such as breast, colorectal, and endometrial cancer. The consumption of whole grains has been associated with a lower risk of cancers, including those affecting the digestive system. Plant-based diets also tend to be low in saturated fats and high in healthy fats like omega-3 fatty acids, which may contribute to a decreased risk of certain cancers, including prostate cancer. Although more research is needed to fully understand the complex relationship between diet and cancer, adopting a plant-based diet is a promising strategy for reducing the risk of this debilitating disease.

THE ROLE OF PHYTONUTRIENTS IN CANCER PREVENTION

Phytonutrients, naturally occurring compounds found in plants, play a crucial role in cancer prevention. These compounds have been extensively researched for their potential anti-cancer properties and have shown promising results in various studies. Phytonutrients are known to possess antioxidant, anti-inflammatory, and anti-microbial properties, all of which contribute to their cancer-fighting abilities. Flavonoids, a type of phytonutrient, have been found to inhibit the growth of cancer cells, induce apoptosis (cell death), and prevent angiogenesis, the process by which tumors develop a blood supply. Other phytonutrients, such as carotenoids and glucosinolates, have also demonstrated anticancer potential. Carotenoids have been shown to reduce the risk of certain types of cancer, including lung, breast, prostate, and colorectal cancer. Glucosinolates, found in cruciferous vegetables like broccoli and cabbage, can help detoxify carcinogens, inhibit the growth of cancer cells, and induce cell death. The consumption of a plant-based diet rich in diverse phytonutrients may be a highly effective strategy for preventing cancer and improving overall health.

EPIDEMIOLOGICAL STUDIES ON DIET AND CANCER INCIDENCE

They have consistently shown a significant association between dietary factors and the risk of developing cancer. These studies provide crucial insights into the impact of diet on cancer incidence rates and offer valuable guidance for preventive and therapeutic interventions. Research has shown that a plant-based diet, rich in fruits, vegetables, whole grains, and legumes, is associated with a reduced risk of various types of cancer, including colorectal, breast, and prostate cancer. This protective effect may be attributed to the high content of bioactive compounds such as antioxidants, phytochemicals, and fiber in plant-based foods, which have been found to suppress cancer cell growth, promote DNA repair, and regulate inflammation. Conversely, diets high in processed meats, red meats, and saturated fats have been consistently associated with an increased risk of cancer. These findings underscore the importance of adopting a healthy and varied diet, emphasizing plant-based foods, to reduce the risk of cancer and promote overall health.

THE ROLE OF PLANT-BASED DIETS IN DIABETES MANAGEMENT

There has been increasing interest in the role of plant-based diets in managing diabetes. Research has shown that adopting a plant-based diet can have numerous benefits for individuals with diabetes, including improved glycemic control, weight loss, and reduced risk of cardiovascular disease. Plant-based diets are typically rich in fiber, vitamins, minerals, and antioxidants, which can help regulate blood sugar levels and promote overall health. A plant-based diet is often low in saturated and trans fats, which are known to increase the risk of insulin resistance and cardiovascular complications in people with diabetes. Plant-based diets have been linked to lower body mass index (BMI) and reduced waist circumference, both of which are important indicators of diabetes management. Studies have also suggested that plant-based diets may decrease the need for medication or insulin in individuals with type 2 diabetes. It is important to note that adopting a plant-based diet alone may not be sufficient for diabetes management, as other lifestyle modifications, such as regular exercise and stress reduction, should also be considered.

BLOOD SUGAR REGULATION THROUGH PLANT-BASED EATING

Blood sugar regulation is a crucial aspect of maintaining overall health and well-being. Consuming a plant-based diet can effectively help in regulating blood sugar levels, preventing the development of various chronic diseases. Plant-based eating focuses on incorporating whole grains, legumes, fruits, vegetables, and nuts, which are nutrient-dense and low in glycemic index. Whole grains, such as quinoa and brown rice, are high in fiber, slowing down the digestion process and preventing spikes in blood sugar. Legumes, such as lentils and chickpeas, are rich in protein and fiber, promoting a gradual and steady rise in blood sugar levels. Fruits and vegetables, especially leafy greens, are not only packed with essential vitamins and minerals but also contain natural sugars that are accompanied by fiber, resulting in a slower and steady increase in blood glucose levels. Nuts, like almonds and walnuts, are excellent sources of healthy fats and fiber, contributing to improved blood sugar control. By adopting a plant-based eating pattern, individuals can effectively regulate blood sugar levels, reduce the risk of diseases like diabetes, and enhance their overall health.

THE ROLE OF DIET IN TYPE 2 DIABETES PREVENTION

Type 2 diabetes has become a highly prevalent condition world-wide, and evidence suggests that diet plays a crucial role in its prevention. Numerous studies have shown that certain dietary patterns, such as a plant-based diet, can significantly reduce the risk of developing type 2 diabetes. A plant-based diet is rich in whole grains, fruits, vegetables, nuts, and legumes, while being low in processed foods, refined grains, and animal products. This dietary approach is high in dietary fiber, antioxidants, and other beneficial compounds that can improve insulin sensitivity, reduce inflammation, and promote weight loss. A plant-based diet has been found to decrease the intake of saturated and trans fats, which are known to contribute to insulin resistance and the development of diabetes. This dietary pattern has shown promising results in improving glycemic control and reducing the need for oral medications or insulin in individuals with established type 2 diabetes. Adopting a plant-based diet can play a significant role in preventing the onset of type 2 diabetes and managing its symptoms in those already diagnosed with the condition.

PLANT-BASED DIETS AND INSULIN SENSITIVITY

An emerging body of research suggests that plant-based diets may play a significant role in improving insulin sensitivity, a key factor in the development and progression of type 2 diabetes. Insulin sensitivity refers to the body's ability to efficiently use insulin to regulate blood sugar levels. Plant-based diets, characterized by high consumption of fruits, vegetables, whole grains, legumes, and nuts, have been found to be rich in fiber and low in saturated fat, both of which are associated with improved insulin sensitivity. The high levels of antioxidants found in plant-based foods may help reduce inflammation and oxidative stress, further contributing to enhanced insulin sensitivity. Several studies have shown that individuals following plant-based diets have a reduced risk of developing type 2 diabetes, as well as improved glycemic control in those with the condition. Plant-based diets have also been associated with weight loss, which is known to be a crucial factor in improving insulin sensitivity. These findings highlight the potential benefits of plant-based diets in promoting insulin sensitivity and preventing or managing type 2 diabetes.

THE ROLE OF PLANT-BASED DIETS IN BONE HEALTH

Plant-based diets have gained popularity in recent years due to their numerous health benefits, but their impact on bone health remains a subject of debate. There is growing evidence that suggests a plant-based diet can provide adequate nutrients for maintaining healthy bones. Plant-based diets are typically rich in fruits and vegetables, which are excellent sources of vitamins and minerals essential for bone health, such as vitamin C, potassium, and magnesium. Plant-based diets are low in animal protein and sodium, which are associated with increased calcium excretion and lower bone mineral density. On the other hand, concerns have been raised about the potential risks associated with plant-based diets, particularly the low intake of certain nutrients, such as calcium and vitamin D, which are crucial for bone health. With careful dietary planning and appropriate supplementation, these concerns can be addressed. A well-balanced plant-based diet can provide the necessary nutrients for maintaining bone health, but individuals following this diet should be mindful of their intake of essential nutrients and consider appropriate supplementation if needed.

CALCIUM SOURCES IN A PLANT-BASED DIET

Calcium is an essential mineral for maintaining strong bones and teeth, as well as supporting proper nerve and muscle function. Many individuals believe that obtaining enough calcium in a plant-based diet can be challenging due to the absence of dairy products, which are commonly associated with high calcium content. A plant-based diet can provide an abundant supply of this vital mineral through various sources. One excellent calcium source in a plant-based diet is dark leafy greens, such as kale, spinach, and collard greens, which are not only low in calories but also rich in calcium. Certain nuts and seeds, including chia seeds, almonds, and sesame seeds, are excellent calcium sources. Plant-based milks fortified with calcium, such as soy milk and almond milk, are also readily available alternatives to cow's milk. Legumes, such as black beans and tofu, offer a considerable amount of calcium. By incorporating these calcium-rich foods into a plant-based diet, individuals can ensure they meet their daily calcium requirements without relying on animal-derived products.

THE ROLE OF VITAMIN D AND MAGNESIUM

Vitamin D, also known as the sunshine vitamin, plays a crucial role in the absorption and utilization of calcium, which is vital for bone health. It also supports the immune system and helps regulate blood pressure. Vitamin D deficiency is becoming increasingly common, especially among individuals following a plant-based diet since vitamin D is primarily found in animal-based products. It is important for individuals relying on plant-based sources to supplement their diet with vitamin D-rich foods like fortified plant-based milks or engage in safe sun exposure. Similarly, magnesium is a mineral that is involved in over 300 biochemical reactions in the body, including energy production, muscle function, and nerve signaling. Plant-based sources of magnesium include green leafy vegetables, nuts, seeds, and whole grains. The low bioavailability of magnesium in plant foods may make supplementation necessary for some individuals. It is crucial to monitor and maintain adequate vitamin D and magnesium levels to ensure optimal overall health, especially for those following a plant-based lifestyle.

PREVENTING OSTEOPOROSIS WITH DIETARY CHOICES

Preventing osteoporosis through dietary choices is a key concern for many individuals, particularly as they age. Osteoporosis, a disease characterized by fragile and weak bones, is a major health problem affecting millions worldwide. Research has shown that dietary choices play a vital role in maintaining bone health and preventing the onset of osteoporosis. The consumption of calcium-rich foods, such as dairy products, leafy green vegetables, and fortified plant-based alternatives, is crucial for optimal bone health. Calcium acts as a building block for bones and helps in maintaining their density. Vitamin D, which facilitates the absorption of calcium, is another essential component in preventing osteoporosis. Sun exposure is a natural source of vitamin D, but dietary sources such as fatty fish, eggs, and fortified cereals are alternate options. Reducing salt intake and maintaining a balanced diet rich in fruits, vegetables, and whole grains can also contribute to healthier bones. Making informed dietary choices can significantly mitigate the risk of osteoporosis and promote lifelong bone health. The adoption of a plant-based diet, which naturally encompasses many of these bone-healthy foods, can further enhance the preventive measures against osteoporosis.

THE ROLE OF PLANT-BASED DIETS IN ALLERGY MANAGEMENT

Plant-based diets have gained considerable attention in recent years due to their potential therapeutic benefits, including their role in managing allergies. Allergies are a common health concern, affecting millions of people worldwide. Current literature suggests that plant-based diets may offer a natural approach to alleviate allergy symptoms and provide relief to those suffering from various allergic conditions. Firstly, plant-based diets are typically rich in anti-inflammatory compounds, such as antioxidants, phytochemicals, and fiber. These components have been shown to reduce inflammation, which is a key factor in the development and severity of allergic reactions. Plant-based diets are often low in saturated fat, which has been linked to increased allergic sensitization. By eliminating animal products from the diet, individuals may reduce their exposure to potential allergenic proteins commonly found in meat and dairy products. It is important to note that individual dietary choices should be made in consultation with a healthcare professional to ensure a well-balanced and nutritionally adequate plant-based diet. Further research is needed to fully explore the mechanisms and potential benefits of plant-based diets in allergy management.

IDENTIFYING AND MANAGING FOOD ALLERGIES

Food allergies occur when the immune system reacts abnormally to certain proteins found in food, leading to a range of symptoms that can vary from mild to life-threatening. In order to properly identify food allergies, individuals may undergo diagnostic tests, including skin prick tests or blood tests, to detect specific antibodies or hypersensitivity reactions. Once a food allergy is confirmed, effective management strategies must be implemented. One of the primary methods of managing food allergies is to avoid consuming the allergen altogether. This can be challenging, especially considering the increasing popularity of plant-based diets that often rely on nuts, soy, or other common allergens. It is crucial for individuals with food allergies, as well as their caregivers and healthcare professionals, to carefully read ingredient labels, thoroughly understand food processing techniques, and communicate effectively to avoid any potential allergen exposure. In certain cases, emergency medications like epinephrine autoinjectors may be prescribed, and individuals should be educated on how to administer these life-saving treatments. Identifying and managing food allergies is essential to ensure the safety and well-being of individuals in the plant-based revolution and beyond.

THE BENEFITS OF AN ELIMINATION DIET

An elimination diet refers to a dietary approach that involves the temporary removal of certain foods or food groups from one's diet. This strategy is often adopted to identify and address potential food sensitivities or allergies, as well as to alleviate symptoms associated with various health conditions. The benefits of an elimination diet are considerable and far-reaching. Firstly, it allows individuals to pinpoint specific foods that may be triggering adverse reactions, such as bloating, digestive issues, or skin problems, thus enabling them to make informed decisions about their diet. By eliminating potential culprits and gradually reintroducing them, individuals can identify the precise triggers and tailor their eating habits accordingly. An elimination diet has shown promising results in the management of chronic conditions like irritable bowel syndrome (IBS), migraines, and autoimmune disorders. This dietary approach has been found to reduce symptoms and improve overall well-being in individuals suffering from these conditions. An elimination diet can promote a more mindful and intentional approach to eating, as individuals become more aware of the impact that different foods have on their bodies. Thus, by adopting an elimination diet, individuals can reap a multitude of benefits and enhance their health and quality of life.

THE ROLE OF PLANT-BASED DIETS IN REDUCING ALLERGIC REACTIONS

Many studies have shown that plant-based diets, which primarily consist of fruits, vegetables, whole grains, legumes, and nuts, are associated with a decreased risk of allergic reactions. This is mainly because plant-based diets are rich in a variety of nutrients, including vitamins, minerals, antioxidants, and phytochemicals, which possess anti-inflammatory and immunomodulating properties. These compounds help to regulate the immune response and reduce the risk of developing allergies. Plant-based diets are naturally low in allergens such as animal proteins, dairy, and gluten, which are common triggers for allergic reactions. The high fiber content in plant-based diets promotes a healthy gut microbiome, which plays a crucial role in immune system regulation. By enhancing gut health, plant-based diets can help prevent the development of allergies and reduce the severity of allergic reactions. Adopting a plant-based diet can have a positive impact on reducing allergic reactions and improving overall health.

CONCLUSION

The plant-based revolution represents a pivotal turning point in our efforts toward sustainability and personal health. It is evident that the rise in popularity of plant-based diets is not merely a passing trend but a strong movement poised to reshape our food systems. As this essay has demonstrated, a plant-based diet offers numerous advantages, both for individuals and the planet. It promotes overall well-being by reducing the risk of chronic diseases and improving the management of existing conditions. It is a more ethical and sustainable approach to food production that alleviates the strain on natural resources and mitigates the adverse environmental effects of animal agriculture. The widespread embrace of plant-based eating poses challenges and opportunities for various stakeholders including farmers, businesses, and policymakers. To ensure its success, we need to foster a supportive infrastructure that enables the accessibility and affordability of plant-based options. Education and awareness campaigns are crucial for dispelling myths and misconceptions surrounding plant-based diets. Embracing a plant-based lifestyle is not only a personal choice but also a collective responsibility towards a healthier and more sustainable future.

SUMMARY OF THE PLANT-BASED REVOLUTION'S IMPACT

The plant-based revolution has had a significant impact on various aspects of society. Firstly, it has revolutionized the way we approach our diets and nutrition. With more and more people adopting plant-based diets, there has been a surge in demand for plant-based food products. This has led to the emergence of a wide range of plant-based alternatives, from meat substitutes to dairy-free products, catering to the needs of vegans and vegetarians. This trend has also prompted restaurants and food chains to include plant-based options on their menus, catering to a broader consumer base. Secondly, the plant-based revolution has also had environmental implications. The expansion of the plant-based industry has resulted in reduced reliance on animal agriculture, which is known for its significant contribution to greenhouse gas emissions and deforestation. By shifting towards plant-based alternatives, individuals are actively contributing to the reduction of their carbon footprint and promoting sustainable practices. The plant-based revolution has sparked conversations about animal welfare and ethical considerations. As more people become aware of the conditions animals face in the food industry, they are opting for plant-based alternatives as a way to minimize harm and promote a more compassionate society. The plant-based revolution has not only impacted our diets and the food industry but also our environment and ethical values.

THE FUTURE OUTLOOK FOR PLANT-BASED DIETS

They appears promising, as the demand for sustainable and environmentally friendly food options continues to grow. With increased awareness of the negative impacts of animal agriculture on climate change and animal welfare, more individuals are adopting a plant-based lifestyle. This shift in dietary habits is not only seen among individuals but also in various industries. An increasing number of restaurants and food companies are offering plant-based options to cater to the growing demand. Technological advancements have allowed for the development of plant-based alternatives that closely resemble animal products in taste and texture. These advancements have contributed to the rising popularity of plant-based diets among a wider range of individuals, including those who previously consumed animal products regularly. Research has highlighted the health benefits associated with plant-based diets, such as lowered risk of chronic diseases and improved overall well-being. As a result, it is likely that plant-based diets will continue to gain traction in the future, offering a sustainable and nutritious alternative for individuals and contributing to a more environmentally conscious society.

FINAL THOUGHTS ON THE ROLE OF INDIVIDUAL CHOICES IN GLOBAL CHANGE

The role of individual choices in global change cannot be understated. As the world faces critical challenges such as climate change and environmental degradation, it is incumbent upon individuals to make conscious decisions that prioritize sustainability and the well-being of the planet. The plant-based revolution represents a powerful example of how personal choices can have significant global impacts. By adopting a plant-based diet, individuals contribute to the mitigation of greenhouse gas emissions, conserve water resources, and alleviate pressures on land and biodiversity. This dietary shift also addresses issues related to public health, including the reduction of obesity and the risk of chronic diseases. It is essential to recognize that individual choices are just one aspect of the solution. Governments, industries, and communities also play pivotal roles in facilitating sustainable practices and shaping policies that incentivize environmentally friendly actions. While individual actions are vital for global change, a collective effort that involves multiple stakeholders is necessary to achieve lasting and widespread impacts. Each person's choices matter, and together, they can drive a significant transformation towards a more sustainable future.

BIBLIOGRAPHY

David Booth. 'The Psychology of Nutrition.' Taylor & Francis, 5/6/2016

Louis Cooper. 'Vegan Meal Prep.' A 30 Days Food Plan. Ready-To-Go Meals and Snacks for a Plant-Based Diet, Independently Published, 1/5/2020

Jackie Kearney. 'Vegan Mock Meat Revolution.' Delicious Plant-based Recipes, Ryland Peters & Small, 12/6/2018

Julie Dare. 'To Eat or Not To Eat Meat.' How Vegetarian Dietary Choices Influence Our Social Lives, Charlotte De Backer, Rowman & Littlefield, 8/20/2019

Richard Crosby. 'Emerging Theories in Health Promotion Practice and Research.' Strategies for Improving Public Health, Ralph J. DiClemente, John Wiley & Sons, 10/15/2002

International Monetary Fund. Fiscal Affairs Dept.. 'Fuel and Food Price Subsidies - Issues and Reform Options.' International Monetary Fund, 8/9/2008

Katherine Kirkwood. 'Alternative Food Politics.' From the Margins to the Mainstream, Michelle Phillipov, Routledge, 12/7/2018

Amy C. Cory. 'Encyclopedia of School Health.' David C. Wiley, SAGE Publications, 8/23/2013

Helen Macbeth. 'Food Preferences and Taste.' Continuity and Change, Berghahn Books, 11/1/1997

Vintage Pen Press. 'Whole Food Plant Based 90 Day Challenge.' Diet Journal and Food Log, CreateSpace Independent Publishing Platform, 10/23/2017

Matthew Willcox. 'The Business of Choice.' Marketing to Consumers' Instincts, Pearson Education, 2/20/2015

David L. Katz. 'Vegetarian Dietary Patterns in the Prevention and Treatment of Disease.' Hana Kahleova, Frontiers Media SA, 8/7/2020

Cristina Santini. 'Plant-Based Food Consumption.' Products, Consumers and Strategies, Giovanna Bertella, Elsevier, 11/3/2023

Brian Watson. 'Vegan Fast Food.' Copycat Burgers, Tacos, Fried Chicken, Pizza, Milkshakes, and More!, Harvard Common Press, 9/27/2022

Ambati Ranga Rao. 'Handbook of Plant-Based Meat Analogs.' Innovation, Technology and Quality, Gokare A. Ravishankar, Elsevier, 5/1/2024

Lutz Grossmann. 'Next-Generation Plant-based Foods.' Design, Production, and Properties, David Julian McClements, Springer Nature, 5/7/2022

Oral Capps. 'Introduction to Agricultural Economics.' John B. Penson, Prentice Hall, 1/1/1996

Virginia Messina. 'Vegan for Life.' Everything You Need to Know to Be Healthy and Fit on a Plant-Based Diet, Jack Norris, Hachette Books, 7/12/2011

James E Houck. 'The Rise of Plant-Based Diets.' : "Why Veganism is Taking Over", Amazon Digital Services LLC - Kdp, 6/29/2023

Kathleen May Kevany. 'Plant-Based Diets for Succulence and Sustainability.' Routledge, 8/15/2019

John McCabe. 'Vegan Myth Vegan Truth.' Obliterating Rumors and Lies about the Earth-saving Diet, Carmania Books, 3/1/2013

Helen Wiseman. 'Phytonutrients.' Andrew Salter, John Wiley & Sons, 4/30/2012

Julieanna Hever. 'The Complete Idiot's Guide to Plant-Based Nutrition.' Penguin, 8/2/2011

Clair Linzey. 'Ethical Vegetarianism and Veganism.' Andrew Linzey, Routledge, 10/25/2018

Robert J. Matthews. 'Ethics, Public Policy, and Agriculture.' Paul B. Thompson, Macmillan, 1/1/1994

Clive Phillips. 'Routledge Handbook of Animal Welfare.' Andrew Knight, Taylor & Francis, 8/15/2022

Jim Mason. 'The Ethics of What We Eat.' Why Our Food Choices Matter, Peter Singer, Harmony/Rodale, 3/20/2007

Pierre Gerber. 'Livestock's Long Shadow.' Environmental Issues and Options, Henning Steinfeld, Food & Agriculture Org., 1/1/2006

Winston J. Craig. 'Vegetarian Nutrition and Wellness.' CRC Press, 6/13/2018

J. D. Wood. 'Nutrition and Climate Change.' Major Issues Confronting the Meat Industry, Nottingham University Press, 4/1/2011

John P. Foreyt. 'Obesity Prevention and Treatment.' A Practical Guide, James M. Rippe, CRC Press, 9/23/2021

Kerrie K. Saunders. 'Vegan Diet as Chronic Disease Prevention.' Lantern Books, 10/1/2003

Raymond J. Cronise. 'Plant-Based Nutrition, 2E.' Julieanna Hever, Penguin, 1/9/2018

Kathy Freston. '72 Reasons to Be Vegan.' Why Plant-Based. Why Now., Gene Stone, Workman Publishing, 3/30/2021

Bob Andrews. 'The Plant-Based Diet Revolution.' 28 Days to a Heathier You, Alan Desmond, Hodder & Stoughton, 1/1/2021

William Shurtleff; Akiko Aoyagi. 'History of Vegetarianism and Veganism Worldwide (1970-2022).' Extensively Annotated Bibliography and Sourcebook, Soyinfo Center, 3/10/2022

Janitha P.D. Wanasundara. 'Sustainable Protein Sources.' Advances for a Healthier Tomorrow, Sudarshan Nadathur, Elsevier, 11/17/2023

Frances Moore Lappé. 'Diet for a Small Planet.' The Book That Started a Revolution in the Way Americans Eat, Random House Publishing Group, 12/8/2010

Meryl Siegal. 'Generation 1.5 in College Composition.' Teaching Academic Writing to U.S.-Educated Learners of ESL, Mark Roberge, Routledge, 2/12/2009

Bob Andrew. 'The Plant-Based Diet Revolution.' 28 days to a happier gut and a healthier you, Alan Desmond, Hodder & Stoughton, 1/7/2021

François Mariotti. 'Vegetarian and Plant-Based Diets in Health and Disease Prevention.' Academic Press, 5/23/2017